HOW
SUCCES

CANDIDA
THE DRUG-FREE WAY

JO DUNBAR

Wellhouse Publishing Ltd

First published in Great Britain in 2003 by
Wellhouse Publishing Ltd
31 Middle Bourne Lane
Lower Bourne
Farnham
Surrey GU10 3NH

Reprinted in 2007

DISCLAIMER

The aim of this book is to provide general information only and should not be treated as a substitute for the medical advice of your doctor or any other health care professional. The publisher and author is not responsible or liable for any diagnosis made by a reader based on the contents of this book. Always consult your doctor if you are in any way concerned about your health.

A catalogue record for this book is available from the British Library

10 Digit ISBN 1-903784-11-5
13 Digit ISBN 978-1-903784-11-2

Printed and bound in Great Britain by
Creative Print & Design (Wales) Ltd., Ebbw Vale

JO DUNBAR

Jo Dunbar was born and brought up in Cape Town, South Africa. Ever since childhood, she has had a fascination with herbal medicines, but thought that herbalism was a medieval concept, until per chance whilst backpacking around England, she discovered the National Institute of Medical Herbalists, who directed her towards the only college of herbal medicine available at the time. After many years of hard study, she now has a thriving herbal medicine practice and retail apothecary in Surrey.

Jo is also involved in supervising dissertation research for BSc degree students at The College of Phytotherapy. She completed her own studies at that institution in 1999, and immediately went on to study a Master of Science degree at the University of Westminster where she focused on Chronic Fatigue Syndrome. Jo can be contacted through The National Institute of Medical Herbalists.

Contents

Introduction

It is amazing how many wide-ranging symptoms may simply be the result of an overgrowth of the yeast-like fungus called *Candida albicans*.

This organism exists in all adult human beings, forming part of the naturally occurring and beneficial flora in the intestines. When there is an overgrowth of this microscopic organism, however, it can lead to many varying and seemingly unrelated symptoms, such as depression or anxiety, abdominal bloating, excessive pre-menstrual symptoms, migraines, feelings of mental fogginess, muscle aches, dandruff and athlete's foot, to name just a few.

Doctors refer to Candida infection as 'intestinal candidiasis' when the overgrowth is limited to the gut, and 'systemic candidiasis' when the overgrowth extends to the rest of the body. Another, older name used by doctors for Candida infection is moniliasis. It is also commonly known as thrush.

Candida overgrowth can become a very serious disorder, and is becoming more and more prevalent in modern times.

Candida infection is a very controversial topic, with complementary practitioners and orthodox doctors hotly debating its very existence. The problem is that, while thrush is a common and well-recognized medical disorder resulting from a Candida yeast infection, unfortunately the more serious condition of a severe yeast overgrowth throughout the body is barely recognized in medical circles. This may be because, frequently, pharmaceutical drugs can actually *cause* the disorder, as we shall see later in this book.

All in Your Head?

Commonly, a patient consulting her doctor with a multiplicity of symptoms is treated for each symptom individually. Unfortunately, rather than the person becoming well again, to her and her doctor's frustration she continues to sink deeper and deeper into ill health.

After a while there may come a time when the sufferer begins to doubt her own sanity, as she may be accused of inventing the illness. She may even be told, 'It's all in your head.' The sufferer is usually certain that something is not right, yet there seems to be no diagnosis to validate her feelings of ill health. This is tremendously upsetting and degrading for a person who is already suffering deeply from a chronic and invasive illness. If this has happened to you, take heart: there *is* a diagnosis *and* a treatment regime for this condition, and people do get better again!

When the yeast population in the gut overgrows, it affects almost every part of the body and causes such a wide range of symptoms that *Candida* has become something of an umbrella term for any collection of symptoms of no identifiable cause. In the past, Candida has been referred to as 'the missing diagnosis'. Because of the wide range of symptoms and the lack of positive diagnostic tests available, this gap provided fertile ground for individuals of limited medical training to hop on the bandwagon and begin 'diagnosing' Candida for almost any condition or illness.

This, understandably, upsets the orthodox medical community, whose ethics demand concrete evidence to prove the existence of disease conditions. Recently, however, although there has been more and more evidence to prove that Candida is a far more widespread problem than was previously believed, most conventional doctors still seem to dispute its existence.

Candida overgrowth is a serious disorder, and it must be recognized that it is a disease of an internal environmental disturbance, and not simply a fungal infection to be treated with anti-fungal medicines. We shall see later in this book how the yeast population is unable to grow out of hand in a healthy body because it is kept in check by the body's immune system and intestinal bacteria. When the body's defence systems break down, however, or when the environment becomes favourable for the yeast to grow, it is able to proliferate and grow out of control wreaking havoc.

A Growing Problem

Candida infection is a big problem. A recent study in the UK showed that 75 per cent of women are affected by vaginal Candida infections, with 40–50 per cent of these women having recurrent episodes of infection.

Although there are thought to be up to 400 species of this yeast, it is specifically *Candida albicans* that I will be discussing in this book. *Candida albicans* accounts for 90 per cent of Candida infections, and is considered the most vicious strain of this particular yeast family. As 'Candida' is the name that most people use when discussing a *Candida albicans* infection, for the sake of convenience I shall simply refer to it as this throughout the book.

How to Use This Book

This book is divided into two parts. Part One goes into some depth in discussing how and why Candida develops. It is important for you to know what causes the overgrowth of yeast, so that these elements may be eliminated before any treatment programme can begin. Part One goes on to discuss in some detail the symptoms of this disorder, and how Candida affects the body.

Part Two focuses on the diagnosis and treatment of Candida. It includes a self-diagnosis chart and a list of recommended laboratory tests required for an accurate diagnosis. This section of the book also has a chapter discussing a thorough treatment programme, and tips on how to adapt your lifestyle comfortably to treating Candida.

Please note that this is a guide to overcoming Candida, and does not by any means act as a substitute for professional treatment. I strongly recommend that you should be treated by a qualified therapist of your choice. A list of professional practitioner bodies is given in the last section of this book.

Let us now move on to understanding the nature of this illness by examining the yeast known as *Candida albicans*.

Part One
The Yeast Environment

Chapter One

The Yeast Environment

Candida albicans is a yeast-like fungus that lives in all of our bodies, and particularly likes to inhabit the moist membranes of the intestines and the vagina, where it feeds off the sugars in our bodies. It is known as a human *commensal* organism, meaning that it naturally lives in our bodies alongside other microscopic bowel flora, without normally causing us any harm.

Until recently, Candida was not thought to contribute towards the host's well-being in any way at all, and was regarded as a harmless parasite and nothing more. However, now it is thought that Candida may actually serve a very interesting purpose. The yeast seems to form a natural protection against exposure to heavy metals, and this is very relevant to the polluted world we live in today. Candida binds heavy metals, so that these toxins can be excreted via the faeces.

Candida does benefit its host, but when the environment becomes conducive to overgrowth, it becomes very dangerous and makes its host very ill. Throughout this book I shall stress that when dealing with Candida you are trying not just to eradicate a yeast overgrowth, but to treat an environmental imbalance. The focus of any treatment programme has to be to rebalance the environment so that the yeast population is put back into its correct proportion.

Candida lives in the gut, alongside the friendly bacteria of the intestines such as *Lactobacillus* and *Bifidobacteria*. These friendly bacteria outnumber the Candida yeast organisms by millions to one, and play a very important role in keeping the Candida population in check and the bowel healthy.

Candida is an interesting organism in that it is able to change forms. It is referred to as a *dimorphic* organism, which literally means that it has 'two shapes and forms'. This is because it has the ability to change from a relatively innocuous yeast form into an invasive fungal form. In its yeast-like form, Candida is a non-invasive, sugar-fermenting organism. It requires oxygen for survival, and in the yeast-like form it competes with the friendly bacteria for oxygen and space. When Candida changes into the fungal form, it no longer requires oxygen for survival and, very importantly, has the ability to develop root-like structures known as rhizoids or mycelia. The mycelia can penetrate the membranes of the intestine, thereby introducing Candida to the bloodstream. As we shall see later, this leads to a whole host of health problems.

When our immune systems are strong and our bodies have not been thrown out of balance by the presence of too much sugar or other imbalances, Candida lives in its yeast form, without impacting negatively on the body. This is partly thanks to the large populations of friendly bacteria which keep the Candida population to a relatively small size by competing vigorously for space, oxygen and food. However, once these control mechanisms are compromised, through illness, drug therapy or poor diet, the yeast changes into its invasive, anaerobic, fungal form.

What Does Yeast Need to Survive?

Candida albicans is a member of the fungus family. In other words it is a mould, and if you think about how easily moulds grow in dark, dank bathrooms, you will get a good idea of the conditions required for a yeast to grow. Yeast thrives in an environment of warmth, darkness and moisture. In order to proliferate, it also needs a constant substrate (source of food) such as sugar to feed on. It is startling how quickly yeast can grow, too. Think also of how amazing it is that large mushrooms can spring up in the forest in a matter of hours, after a warm, damp night. These mushrooms seem to come from nowhere, and yet in a matter of hours have produced large fungal bodies made up of billions of cells. The fungus was already there, underground, but the environmental conditions weren't conducive for mushroom growth. As soon as the conditions were right, the fungus's ability to produce billions of cells in a matter of hours is astonishing. Yeast can grow at a phenomenal speed, given the right environment.

So what we are talking about is not a matter of the fungus being the problem. Fungal spores are everywhere; it is only when the conditions are right for the fungus's proliferation that problems can arise. We have Candida yeast living in our bodies all the time, but we don't suffer from an overgrowth unless conditions allow that to happen.

What we are talking about is an environmental issue. Rebalance the environment, and your problem will be resolved. Getting rid of mould in a bathroom has nothing to do with using a mould spray. If you leave the bathroom as a dark and moist environment, you can use all the bottles of anti-mould spray you like; the mould will simply return within a matter of days. However, if you change the environment and make it less hospitable to the mould by improving the natural daylight and air-flow to eliminate the dampness, you will find that the mould does not grow anymore. Using the anti-mould spray will speed up the eradication of the mould, but anti-mould spray by itself simply cannot completely eradicate the problem. In much the same way, you will never eliminate Candida simply by using anti-fungal medications. You *must* change your internal environment.

A Matter of Conservation

In order to understand why treating Candida has very little to do with anti-fungal treatment, and everything to do with rebalancing the internal environment, let us examine some of the laws of life.

A basic law of life is the quest for survival. All organisms will take whatever opportunity there is in order to survive and thrive. It is a matter of taking advantage of a gap in the market of life. The balance of life is mediated between the fact that all living organisms have the potential to expand their populations indefinitely, and the restrictions placed on these populations by their natural enemies. If a population of organisms can expand at the expense of other organisms, they will do so. Such is the harsh reality of life, and we can see this even in our carefully manipulated human world. All organisms will exploit their environment, and are kept in check only by their natural enemies. Every living organism has natural enemies which keep the population numbers at a sustainable balance for the good of the whole. If you take these enemies away, however, there is nothing to restrict the growth of the expanding population. It grows and feeds voraciously on the surrounding environment and eventually depletes the food supplies.

In order to continue to grow, there is nothing else for the population to do but to spread further in search of more food and space to support itself. The most successful survivors are those which can adapt to new environments, or change the environment to suit their requirements for life. Candida is kept in check by its competitors the friendly intestinal bacteria and by its natural enemy, the immune system. If you change this balance by removing the bacteria and depleting your immune system, and add to this by increasing Candida's food supply in the form of sugars, the population will explode.

Anyone who has made wine can bear testament to the startling speed at which yeast can grow in the presence of sugars. This is what can happen in the body, given the right conditions, and the modern Western lifestyle provides just such perfect conditions.

It is easy to see how our bodies have the potential to provide the correct environment for a Candida population explosion. Our bodies are warm and moist, and sugars we digest feed the Candida yeast organisms. But why doesn't everybody have a Candida problem? The answer is the yeast's natural enemies as mentioned, the friendly bacteria which compete with Candida for space and food, and also our immune system, which acts as a scavenger and gobbles up any escapees.

French physicians describe treating the internal environment as treating the *terraine*. You can compare your health to a garden. If the soil is poor and without nourishment, then plant growth will not be robust. A garden treated with pesticides tends to kill off *all* insects, even normally beneficial ones, and thus the garden is vulnerable to insect damage (unless you keep spraying) because it lacks the natural friendly insect predators to fight off the pests. In order to grow a productive garden, we nourish the soil with compost and manure, and we allow a natural ecosystem to develop where a biodiversity of insects keep their populations in a natural balance within the garden. In this way we develop a sustainable garden.

Holistic practitioners treat illness in the same way. We treat the terraine or the internal environment. The key to treating Candida successfully is to treat the environment. Good health will follow naturally.

Summary

- Candida is a yeast-like fungus which naturally lives in the bodies of all adult humans.
- *Candida albicans* is a dimorphic organism with the ability to change from the yeast form into the invasive fungal form.
- Candida needs warmth, darkness, moisture and food to survive.
- The Candida population is kept in check by the immune system and friendly gut bacteria.
- The Candida population needs a lack of enemies and plentiful supply of food to expand.

The conditions of food, lack of competitors and a depleted immune system required for the Candida population to expand and become disease-producing seem simple. On deeper investigation, however, there are many mechanisms which give us the tendency to develop the environment required for Candida overgrowth. In the following chapters we shall investigate these mechanisms more deeply, so that they can be understood and dealt with by the treatment programme outlined in Part Two.

ChapterTwo

Population Explosion

Why does Candida become a problem? We all have Candida living in our bodies, and yet it seems that certain people are more susceptible than others to Candida becoming a real problem. Once again, all the reasons for overgrowth point towards an internal environmental imbalance, rather than simply a Candida infection.

In the previous chapter we looked at the basic requirements of life for a yeast organism and saw that, to survive, the Candida yeast needs warmth, moisture and darkness. In order for the fungal population to explode, Candida requires a plentiful supply of food, a lack of their natural competitors (the friendly intestinal bacteria), and a depleted natural enemy (the host's immune system). Other imbalances, as we shall see later, are an added bonus for the Candida.

Warmth, moisture and darkness are obviously a part of our biological make-up. The yeast lives in the warm and moist mucous membranes of our bodies, and there is nothing we can do about that. However, those are only the conditions required for its *survival*. The conditions which allow for an overabundance of the Candida population, such as loss of the friendly bacteria, a depleted immune system, hormonal imbalances and high blood sugar levels are avoidable. However, when these conditions arise, there is very little to stop a Candida population explosion.

Candida is a very complicated disorder. Like many modern diseases, a Candida overgrowth seems to have multiple causes. Many studies have noted that *Candida albicans* can be found on vaginal swabs from women who are not suffering from the symptoms of a Candida infection. This clearly suggests that Candida in itself is not the problem. Rather, it demonstrates that changes in the vaginal environment are required before the fungus can exert its adverse effects.

As well as the fact that a wide diversity of factors can result in an overgrowth of the organism, it is quite likely that not all of these conditions will apply directly in your particular case. However, almost all of the conditions which have this effect relate directly to our modern Western lifestyle. Let us now look more closely at the factors that may contribute towards a yeast overgrowth in our bodies.

The Five Major Causes of Candida Overgrowth

1. A depletion of the friendly bacteria
2. A breakdown of our natural defence system the immune system
3. A hormonal imbalance
4. High blood sugar levels, caused either by diet, stress or diabetes
5. Drug therapy

The Friendly Bacteria

Within our intestines lives a huge colony of beneficial bacterial micro-organisms, as well as the less friendly organisms such as Candida yeast, *E. coli* and *Streptococci* bacteria. There are many different species of bacteria, but the two most beneficial and well-studied bacteria are the *Lactobacilli* and *Bifidobacteria*. These are the *probiotics* which you can buy at a chemist's or health food store. These friendly bacteria are essential in our fight against Candida, and for our general health.

All the micro-organisms that live in the digestive tract are known as 'commensal organisms'. They normally live in our bodies without actually causing any harm when their populations are kept in the correct proportions.

The digestive tract extends from the mouth to the anus, but the commensal organisms live primarily in the stomach, small intestine and large intestine. The digestive tract becomes increasingly devoid of oxygen as it descends towards the anus, and the types of bacteria present reflect the amount of oxygen available. The stomach has the smallest population of organisms (fewer than 100 organisms per gram of contents), being very inhospitable to life due to its extremely high-acid environment and rapid emptying actions. The small intestine is an alkaline environment and still has fairly high levels of oxygen. These are conditions that suit the *Lactobacilli* bacteria, as well as Candida when it is in its yeast form. Here we see the population of commensals increasing to between 10,000 and 1,000,000 organisms per gram of contents. In the large intestine the environment has almost no oxygen, and although there are small populations of *Lactobacilli*, it is the *Bifidobacteria* that dominate here. The large intestine has a very slow pattern of movement, making it conducive for the establishment of bacterial populations, and here we find one thousand billion organisms per gram of contents. Indeed, our digestive system is so full of bacteria that between 30 and 50 per cent of the faecal weight is made up of dead bacteria!

Lactobacilli and *Bifidobacteria* perform the very important task of keeping the other bacteria and yeast micro-organism populations in check through vigorous competition for space, oxygen and food. These friendly bacteria establish themselves in every possible available space within the intestine, and essentially out-compete other organisms such as Candida. In doing so they deny the less friendly organisms the necessary requirements to be able to thrive. Therefore the Candida population cannot expand to disease-producing proportions. These friendly bacteria also produce organic acids, which have the effect of making the environment less hospitable for the Candida, because Candida likes an alkaline environment.

These friendly bacteria are vital to our health and perform various important functions such as stimulating our immune system, producing certain vitamins and, very importantly, keeping other organism populations in check by vigorously competing for space, food and oxygen. In other words, *Lactobacilli* and *Bifidobacteria* are the major warriors against a Candida overgrowth.

Protection Against Dysbiosis

Because the friendly bacteria compete so successfully against the Candida yeast for food and space, the Candida yeast population is normally very much smaller compared to the beneficial bacterial population. Dysbiosis occurs in the digestive system when an imbalance of gut flora allows the unfriendly bacteria and yeast populations to dominate, leading to adverse health effects.

When Candida is allowed to dominate the gut environment, it is able to transform into the fungal form, where it develops root-like mycelia that can penetrate the gut wall and enter the bloodstream. The potential to cause great harm to the body is enormous, especially when the immune system is weak. Essentially, this is exactly what happens in the disorder known as Candida.

How Does a Dysbiosis Occur?

In the case of Candida, dysbiosis occurs usually through the over-use of antibiotics.

Antibiotics have revolutionized our armoury against bacterial infection and, I am sure, we all gratefully acknowledge that they have saved millions of lives, possibly even our own. Probably due to their astounding success, they have until very recently become over-prescribed by well-meaning doctors for non-life-threatening bacterial infections such as the common cold or acne. As a result, most of us have probably had numerous unnecessary courses of antibiotics during our lives, and now we are counting the cost.

Until recently it was not really understood that these wonder drugs could have a detrimental effect on our health but they do. A typical story can be related through the experience of a patient of mine.

Barry developed a persistent sore throat and was given a course of antibiotics to treat it. The sore throat did not resolve, and his doctor prescribed another course of stronger antibiotics. Barry's throat became worse, and eventually it became so badly swollen that he could barely breathe. Finally he was admitted to hospital, given intravenous antibiotics and eventually his sore throat resolved. The sore throat 'cure' was temporary, but the antibiotics had annihilated the friendly bacterial population in his gut. When I met Barry he had developed thrush and his sore throat had recurred. Astonishingly, his doctor had offered to re-prescribe the first batch of antibiotics. At this point Barry decided to opt for natural treatment. Fortunately his Candida overgrowth was still in its infancy and was quickly cured by a course of probiotics, which replenished the friendly bacterial population in his digestive system. An immune tonic sorted out his sore throat, and he had no further need for medication.

Antibiotics are one of the major contributors to dysbiosis and Candida overgrowth. This is what happens.

Antibiotics will kill the disease-causing bacteria, but they will also kill all the bacteria in the body, including the friendly bacteria residing in our intestines. Antibiotics have a devastating effect on the friendly bacterial populations. Very few of these friendly bacteria survive. Perversely, more of the unfriendly bacteria manage to survive than the friendly bacteria. Moreover, yeasts such as *Candida albicans* are not at all affected by antibiotics, and immediately take advantage of the disaster suffered by the friendly bacteria. The unfriendly bacterial populations, which are normally kept in check by the friendly bacteria, also expand at a faster rate than the friendly bacterial populations, and are able also to take advantage of the space that has become available. So, without its natural enemy to compete with, Candida proliferates and 'fills the gap' by occupying every niche that has suddenly become available.

Once the Candida yeast population is allowed to expand, it changes into the fungal form. The fungal form of Candida does not require oxygen for survival, and this allows it to migrate into the large intestine and also the bloodstream. In the fungal form, it enters the bloodstream by producing the mycelia which penetrate the lining of the gut, leading to a leaky gut, and allowing the Candida to escape into the bloodstream and the whole body. So the Candida has changed from a well-controlled, oxygen-dependent yeast into the rampant fungal form with the ability to migrate into parts of the body which were previously inhospitable to the organism. Other unfriendly bacteria further promote the invasion of Candida into the bloodstream by causing inflammation of the gut lining, which contributes to a leaky gut and all the problems associated with such a condition.

Don't be fooled into believing that it is only the antibiotic pills that cause this severe disruption. I have a patient who had a student job working at the fish counter in a supermarket. Every evening he had to clean the steel fish trays with a powerful antibacterial disinfectant solution. This potent substance leached into his body via the skin on his hands, and led to a severe and prolonged systemic Candida attack.

Major Causes of Dysbiosis
- antibiotics
- gastric infection
- gastric surgery

Less Common Causes of Dysbiosis
- starvation, anorexia or nutritional deficiency
- Irritable Bowel Syndrome

Other Benefits of Probiotics

Another function of the friendly bacteria is to prime the immune system. *Lactobacilli* and *Bifidobacteria* stimulate the development of the immune system in newborn babies, and continue to modulate the immune system throughout our lives. In fact they are so effective at improving the immune response that probiotics have been referred to as the third element of the immune system, and scientists are using these microbes therapeutically to improve the immune response in HIV-infected children, with very positive results.

The action of probiotics has been described as having the effect of 'turning the immune system on again', and helping the immune system do what it wants to do in terms of attacking assailants. As with Candida, we all have cancer cells in our bodies, but those of us with good immune systems do not go on to develop cancer because the cells of our immune systems destroy these rogue cells. Recent studies have suggested that probiotics may have such a stimulating effect on the immune system that they may even have possible anti-tumour actions.

Another protective action that the probiotics exert is antibiotic production. *Lactobacilli* such as *Lactobacillus acidophilus* produce certain substances that exert inhibitory effects against both foreign bacteria and *Candida albicans*. There is little evidence to suggest that *Bifidobacteria* produce antibiotics, but they also seem to exert averse effects on pathogens (disease-forming microbes) such as Candida.

The beneficial bacteria also stimulate the digestion and absorption of nutrients. Nutrients which are difficult to absorb, such as the milk sugar lactose, are more easily digested because these beneficial bacteria produce the enzyme 'lactase', which breaks the sugar down into more easily digestible parts. Friendly bacteria also help to prevent malnutrition by actually synthesizing vitamins such as Folic acid and certain B vitamins, and by improving mineral availability. Of particular importance is that the friendly bacteria produce the B vitamin Biotin, which helps to block yeast overgrowth.

The probiotics also have the effect of slowing the passage of food through the stomach, so that the food has the opportunity to become well digested by stomach acids. At the same time, this stimulates intestinal movement and prevents constipation.

Summary

- The commensal organism population is made up of both beneficial and disease-producing organisms.
- The population distribution is determined by oxygen supply, gut movement and the acid/alkali balance.
- When friendly bacterial populations are wiped out, the niche is filled by Candida and less beneficial bacteria.
- Candida changes from the yeast form into the fungal form and penetrates the gut wall with mycelia, causing a leaky gut. This provides passage for the Candida to migrate into other parts of the body.
- The friendly bacteria (probiotics) of the digestive system keep the Candida population in check.
- Probiotics also stimulate the immune system, stimulate the digestion and synthesis of nutrients, and influence gut movement.

Chapter Three

Your Body's Defence System

Although many doctors have difficulty in accepting that Candida may be causing disease in a perfectly healthy-looking person, the medical establishment is in agreement that systemic Candida is a major problem in certain immune-deficient disease conditions such as AIDS. Other conditions where one might commonly find Candida infection affecting the whole body include Chronic Fatigue Syndrome (also known as ME), cancer and certain other chronic illnesses. Immune-suppression therapy, used after an organ transplant operation or to treat auto-immune diseases, also (as its name suggests) suppresses our immune system. Inflammatory conditions such as arthritis or asthma are treated with corticosteroids, which also have the effect of suppressing the immune system.

What do all these disorders have in common? Quite simply, the immune system has either been deliberately suppressed with medications, or long-term illness has placed the immune system under such duress that it is quite unable to mount any further attacks against assailants. Alternatively, the body is infected with a micro-organism which specifically destroys the immune system, as in AIDS. However, not everyone who develops Candida is suffering from these severe disorders. Some people simply exhaust their bodies (and immune systems) through their busy lifestyles.

Jed's Story
I have a male patient who is just this sort of person. If you looked at him, you would never guess there was anything wrong with him. He appears to be a strong, healthy and robust man in his mid-thirties, yet he has struggled to beat Candida for some time. The problem with Jed was that he has really lived life to the full. He got onto the career ladder and did very well in his line of work, and was consequently given more and more responsibility. As a result, he worked very long hours. Keen not to miss out on life, he would race off to the gym after work and then, whenever he could, he would be out and about having fun. In

among this frantic lifestyle, he certainly did not have time to prepare proper meals for himself, so he ate high-carbohydrate foods and coffee on the run, and then calmed down in the pub with a few beers.

Jed was burning his body out with so much stress and activity, and not nourishing it with a good diet. In fact, his diet contributed to his ill health. Whenever Jed became ill he would soldier on regardless, because he thought he could fight through the illness. In the end he became so ill that he simply did not recover. He lay in bed for weeks. At this stage Jed became my patient and, following tests, I diagnosed Candida.

Jed's recovery has been a slow process. He has recognized that his problem lay in his lifestyle, and has moderated his life and diet significantly. His immune resistance is much improved and his symptoms of Candida have almost vanished, but he does have to be very careful not to over-extend himself, because if he does, his symptoms will recur.

How Our Immune System Works

Our immune system can be likened to our own personal army, which defends us against detrimental invading foreign organisms and particles. The immune system is complicated, made up of two distinct lines of defence.

The first line of defence comprises physical barriers including the skin and the mucous membranes of the lungs, gastro-intestinal tract and vaginal tract, the mucous in our lungs, and many other systems. This first line of defence physically resists micro-organism invasion into the internal environment of the body.

The second line of defence is much more complicated, and this takes place within the bloodstream.

Some people regard the beneficial flora which reside in our intestines as our third line of defence. These friendly bacteria have been shown, as mentioned in Chapter Two, to prime the immune system in newborn babies.

Since Candida naturally resides in our digestive tract, let us look at the first line of defence as it exists in the gut.

The First Line of Defence
First of all, try to imagine your body as a tube within a tube. The digestive tract can be seen as the inner tube, which runs from the mouth to

the anus without any break. Essentially, because this inner tube is uninterrupted and runs from mouth to anus, it can be seen as a barrier against our external environment, and serves as an excellent first line of defence.

The contents of the gut, or inner tube, are made up primarily of undigested food particles and medicines (in the small intestine), and of digested food particles and faecal matter (in the large intestine). These substances are seen by the body as members of the external environment.

The body's 'outer tube' is made up of the contents of our delicately balanced internal environment, such as the circulatory system, the internal organs, the tissue cells and the finely tuned chemical balance of fluids bathing these cells.

All the contents of the gut are potentially dangerous to the internal environment of the body. Were the contents of the external environment allowed to enter the internal environment without censure, they would cause us great illness either through microbial or toxin invasion. Before some of these constituents are allowed to enter the internal environment of the body, they must first be digested by our enzyme system, and then passed through the liver for toxin removal.

The inner tube, or digestive tract, is lined with a thin mucous membrane which acts as a frontier zone, keeping the external environment separate from the internal environment. It is made up of tiny gateways which selectively allow only digested food particles and medications to enter the internal environment. If this barrier were to become too permeable, as with a 'leaky gut', it would allow undigested food particles and toxins to enter the bloodstream and the internal environment.

The walls of the small intestine are lined with patches of immune tissue known as MALT cells. These MALT cells act to protect the body against invasion from microbes and other foreign materials. Bear in mind that the friendly bacteria and the Candida yeast live within the environment of the small intestine (inner tube). Should the friendly bacteria be killed, by antibiotics for instance, the Candida population has no enemies within the inner tube. It is then free to change into its fungal form and grow the mycelia which penetrate the lining of the inner tube. This is essentially what is known as 'leaky gut syndrome'. The mycelia produce whopping great holes in the first line of defence, which allow undigested food particles and toxins to enter the bloodstream. This invariably leads to many of the symptoms associated with Candida food allergies, muscle ache, loss of mental clarity, etc. – because the body is being poisoned. It also means that the Candida organism has entered the internal environment. Remember that in its fungal form, the Candida no longer requires oxygen to live, so it is quite happy to expand its population beyond the boundaries of the oxygenated gut.

The Second Line of Defence

Should a foreign invader manage to escape into the internal environment, it will encounter the formidable second line of defence, the white blood cells of our immune system. Lymphocytes are immune-regulating cells which circulate in the bloodstream and belong to the family of white blood cells. The lymphocytes themselves are divided into two arms of defence. All lymphocytes are produced in the bone marrow, but they migrate to different sites in the body to become activated:

- Lymphocytes that migrate to the thymus gland (located beneath the breast bone) become known as T-cells.
- Other lymphocytes that become activated in the bone marrow are referred to as B-cells.

T-cells attack foreign invaders directly. This form of immune function is called *cell-mediated immunity*. When the T-cells discover rogue cancer cells or invaders such as Candida, they immediately mount an attack and kill the offender. However, people with a lowered immune response as a result of either illness, medication or lifestyle cannot respond effectively enough. This is when they become susceptible to disease. Research has shown that people are particularly susceptible to Candida invasion when the cell-mediated arm of the immune system is suppressed. When the immune system can no longer defend the internal environment against invading fungi such as Candida, the fungus has *carte blanche* to invade the body as it pleases.

The B-cells, for their part, secrete specific antibodies against particular invaders such as micro-organisms or even proteins. This response is known as *humoral immunity*. When undigested food particles or Candida enter the bloodstream via a leaky gut, the body recognizes these as foreign invaders. The B-cells also have a memory so that, every time a particular food substance or yeast is presented to the immune system in the blood, the B-cells will immediately begin to secrete antibodies against the offender. This is how food and yeast allergies develop, as a reaction by the body to what it recognizes as foreign invaders.

Why Candida Loves Stress

Our bodies are designed to cope with stress, but only short-term stress. When we face either a physical, mental or emotional stress, our adrenal glands, which are situated on top of our kidneys, pump out the hormone *cortisol*.

Cortisol is the body's natural version of the medicines known as corticosteroids. Cortisol has an anti-inflammatory action, and it is for this reason that corticosteroid therapy, the synthesized version of cortisol, is of such value in inflammatory conditions such as asthma or arthritis.

Stress elicits a 'fight or flight' response in humans, and both of these reactions require a massive output of energy in order to help us escape or deal successfully with potentially dangerous situations. Cortisol is one of the hormones that helps the body to react success-fully to stressful situations by converting stored energy, in the form of fat, into available energy in the form of blood sugar. This is a natural and life-saving mechanism, which we are provided with in order to survive the occasional short-term stressful events that we inevitably come across. However, in the 21st century we are rarely exposed to the same kind of life-threatening situations our ancestors were. Yet we impose more artificial stressors on our bodies: running to catch a train, rushing to meet deadlines, fighting through divorce proceed-ings, surviving redundancy, etc. Living these very stressed lives, our cortisol output far exceeds that which is natural for us, and this is where the problem sets in.

In the long term, too much cortisol has the effect of suppressing cellular immunity. Remember that the white blood cells are divided into two arms, which promote either cellular or humoral immunity. These two arms are normally held in balance, as if they were a per-fectly balanced pair of scales. An excess of cortisol has the effect of depressing cellular immunity, and promoting humoral immunity. In doing so, the immune system scales are tipped, with cellular immu-nity being depressed and humoral immunity accentuated.

What does this mean? This means that the killer activity of the T-cells (cellular immunity) is suppressed so that the body is handicapped in its fight against Candida invasion. It also means that the B-cells (humoral immunity) are working overtime, secreting antibodies and setting up allergic and intolerant reactions to everything they believe is foreign to the internal environment. This is really what an allergic response is all about. The humoral arm of the immune system is over-reacting to certain stimuli. So we have cellular immunity under-reacting to Candida invasion, and humoral immunity over-reacting to Candida and food invasion into the internal environment.

The ultimate outcome of this scenario is that the body can eventually become so confused that the immune system turns to attack the very body that it should be protecting. The immune system actually attacks its own tissues as well as foreign invaders. This is what is referred to as an *auto-immune disease*. Several studies have noted a strong link between systemic Candida and auto-immune diseases, especially those involving the thyroid gland.

The situation gets even worse, however. Cortisol not only has the effect of suppressing the immune system so that it is unable to fight the Candida effectively, but normally it helps us cope with stress by increasing the blood sugar output. Cortisol releases blood sugar by converting fat and protein into glucose. This essentially means that the enfeebled immune response allows the Candida to gatecrash the bloodstream of the internal environment, and then provides the Candida with its favourite food – a nice constant supply of sugar in the blood.

A typical case scenario might go something like this:

Penny has a stressful job and an extremely busy lifestyle. She has no time to cook, so she eats fast food on the run and often eats a chocolate bar for the sugar boost of energy. This constant state of stress results in an increased release of cortisol, which depresses her immune system, and there are precious few nutrients available from her diet to compensate for this added pressure.

Of course, Penny becomes ill. She develops a cold. She tries to fight it off, but eventually decides to try a course of antibiotics. Her friendly gut bacteria are wiped out, and the Candida population is left a clear run to expand. The Candida yeast no longer has bacteria to compete with and is thus able to take advantage of the gap and change into its fungal form. The Candida fungus then penetrates Penny's gut lining and gains access to her bloodstream, along with undigested food particles.

Penny's immune system is already depleted, you remember, but now it is confronted with an invader Candida. So the T-cells mount an attack against the fungus, but the Candida has no enemies in the gut and is very strong. The T-cells are already weakened by the hormonal effects of cortisol as well as being under pressure to cope with clearing millions of bacteria and viruses each day. Now the T-cells have the added pressure of having to mount an attack against the fungal invasion.

In the mean time, food constantly escapes through the holes in the gut wall, so the B-cells are continually confronted with antigens against which they must secrete protective antibodies. Penny starts to develop food intolerances, and becomes even more ill. Her immune system is exhausted, while the Candida thrives.

What Can We Do?

Hold in your mind's eye that the immune system is much like a pair of scales which are, ideally, in a natural balance. We do not constantly have the same output of immune response throughout our 24-hour day. During the day we find that the humoral arm dominates the scene, and at night, during periods of rest, the cellular immune system kicks into action. Studies have shown that sleep deprivation adversely affects the cellular immune system, making it less effective. It makes sense, therefore, to postulate that plenty of rest will have a positive effect on our immunity, by boosting the depleted cellular immune arm and giving the overactive humoral arm a break. Haven't you noticed how much more easily you become ill when you haven't rested enough?

Please understand that it is not cortisol which is the problem here. It is our stressful environment, which predisposes us to secreting too much cortisol over too long a period of time.

A more difficult question arises when we question what to do about people who rely on corticosteroid therapy for the treatment of inflammatory conditions. Corticosteroids are very commonly prescribed for conditions such as asthma, arthritis and certain bowel diseases. Even the topical steroid cremes used to control eczema in children, or the steroids in asthma inhalers, leach into the body and have similar detrimental effects.

In fact, many of these diseases can be very successfully treated using natural medicine. If corticosteroid therapy is causing your overgrowth of Candida, then you have a serious enough problem to warrant investigating alternative and more natural methods for treating the problem.

Of primary importance is rebalancing and restoring the immune system. The immune system, the adrenal glands and the nervous system all urgently need to be given a helping hand, and this can be achieved through a comprehensive treatment programme, as outlined in Part Two. This will ideally include the use of herbal medicines, acupuncture, homeopathy and nutritional therapy. Of course, rest and recovery are extremely important and, as well as making sure that you get enough good-quality sleep, it can be very beneficial to take up some relaxation activities such as yoga, tai chi, meditation or a regular aromatherapy massage.

All of these therapies and methods focus on rebalancing the whole person. We are not just killing the fungus, we are aiming for a cure. To do so we need to treat the underlying cause of the illness, so we need holistic (whole-person) treatment.

Summary: Causes of Poor Immunity

- stress
- poor nutrition
- immune-suppressive diseases such as HIV, Chronic Fatigue Syndrome
- immuno-suppressive drug therapy for organ transplants and auto-immune diseases
- chemotherapy for cancer treatment
- long-term or recurrent steroid therapy
- long-term or repeated antibiotic therapy
- environmental antibiotics found in meat, fish, eggs and dairy products

Chapter Four

The Hormonal Connection

It has long been noted that people who are otherwise healthy, but also suffer from Candida infections or recurrent thrush, are predominantly women. The National Candida Society in Britain notes from their surveys that at least 60 per cent of sufferers are women, with 20 per cent being men and 20 per cent children. Moreover, these women tend to suffer at times of their lives when their hormone levels are peaking. Most women prone to Candida or vaginal thrush tend to succumb to it just before their period, or during pregnancy. Other women have noticed that they have become more prone to it while on the contraceptive pill or taking Hormone Replacement Therapy. So why is it that women suffer from Candida significantly more than other members of our population?

Why Candida disproportionately affects women is still not clear. There is some interesting research available, but at the moment we are still not sure *exactly* why it affects predominately women.

What we *do* know is that it has nothing to do with the female genital area being darker, warmer or moister than the male genital area, and nor does it mean that women are less clean than men. Numerous studies note that women routinely have Candida yeast on their vaginal swabs without suffering from any symptoms of thrush. This once again suggests an environmental imbalance. But what is it that changes the vaginal conditions from inhospitable to those which encourage the yeast to proliferate? Research clearly points to the female hormones.

The two major hormones in the female cycle are progesterone and oestrogen, which tend to dominate at different times during the monthly cycle, but both have peaks during the pre-menstrual phase of the cycle the time when many women succumb to thrush.

Other factors may also influence the ability of Candida yeast to proliferate. The vagina and vulva of the female genital tract are naturally slightly acidic, as opposed the male genital tract, which is predominately alkaline. The acidity of the female tract is important in that it

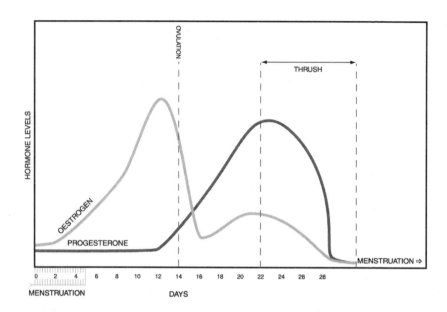

provides the correct environment for the protective bacteria to live in. When the acid/alkaline balance changes to become more alkaline, the naturally protective acid-loving bacteria die, and leave space for opportunistic infections such as Candida to grow.

A study conducted at an American University looked at what happens to the vaginal mucous membrane layer, and the natural bacteria which reside there, when synthesized progesterone is introduced to the body. They noted that the progesterone produced a false state of reduced oestrogen, which reduced the numbers of acid-loving *Lactobacillus* bacteria and decreased the thickness of the membrane layer. This made the women more prone to infection by Candida yeast organisms. Although all women seem to house Candida within their genital tract, a false state of high progesterone and low oestrogen had the effect of making the women more susceptible to Candida infection.

This is in contrast to a study conducted at another American University, which concluded that, while progesterone does not contribute at all towards Candida overgrowth, high levels of oestrogen reduce the vaginal membrane's ability to inhibit Candida growth. Another study noted that synthesized oestrogen encourages the growth of *Candida albicans*, as well as making the Candida more resistant to anti-fungal medication. Finally, an Australian doctor found that post-menopausal women using oestrogen supplements (HRT) were significantly more prone to Candida infection. He has suggested that oestrogen increases the production of glycogen, which provides a sweet substance for the Candida to feed off.

What have all these studies in common with pregnancy, the hormonal status of a pre-menstrual woman, and women taking the Pill or Hormone Replacement Therapy?

Elevated Levels of Oestrogen and Progesterone

The situation looks confusing, but what does seem to be clear is that an overgrowth of Candida cannot simply be related to an overabundance of either one or other hormone, but rather to an imbalance within the female hormonal system.

Hormones and hormonal receptors work according to a lock-and-key system. Hormonal receptors are found throughout the body, and can initiate action once the specific hormone that acts as the key fits into a receptor and 'turns the lock'. Without the receptors, the hormone cannot express its potential action. The National Candida Society suggests that in some cases, oestrogen receptors may be blocked (by unnatural oestrogens), leading to a *relative* increase in progesterone. In other words, a hormone imbalance results, with the progesterone activity being relatively higher than normal and that this contributes to the Candida problem. Several members of the National Candida Society have confirmed this theory by noting that their Candida symptoms become significantly worse after taking progesterone supplements, even in the form of 'natural' progesterone cream. Other writers on the subject agree that neither of the two major female hormones is to blame for Candida overgrowth, but that an imbalance between the two causes symptoms to occur.

It is important to realize that, like cortisol, the sex hormones are also part of the group of steroid hormones. So when we take in unnatural quantities of sex hormones such as oestrogen or progesterone, we unwittingly increase our steroid load which will disrupt the immune system.

What Causes Hormone Imbalances?
When taking the research data and surveys into account, it seems likely that a hormonal imbalance results from the excessive intake

of unnatural hormones, which may block hormonal receptor sites, thus leading to an imbalance in the delicately tuned hormonal system. It is this that encourages yeast to proliferate.

Hormone-imbalance Triggers
- Antibiotics and steroid therapy
- Feminine hygiene products
- Sexual intercourse
- Hormone therapy HRT, the Pill, 'natural' progesterone cream
- Environmental hormones found in meat, eggs, milk and dairy products
- Hormonal changes puberty, pregnancy, the menopause, pre-menstrual changes

Antibiotics and Steroid Therapy
Apart from killing off the friendly gut bacteria and depressing the immune system, medicines such as antibiotics and corticosteroids can play yet another role in encouraging yeast overgrowth.

Oestrogen is formed in the ovaries and the adrenal glands. During the menstruating years, the adrenal glands barely contribute towards oestrogen levels, but after the menopause this contribution becomes very significant for general health reasons.

Steroids mimic the cortisol produced in our adrenal glands. Taking steroids supresses (atrophies) these glands because their work is being done for them. Thus they can fail to produce the necessary oestrogen, and this can lead to an imbalance, with progesterone dominating.

Corticosteroid therapy is routinely used for conditions such as arthritis. Women usually develop arthritis as they become more mature, which just happens to coincide with the menopausal years and women's reliance on adrenal oestrogen supplies.

Many women feel cautious about taking antibiotics, because they know that if they do, they may develop thrush. Broad-spectrum antibiotics kill all the bacteria of the body, including the friendly bacteria of the gut and vaginal area, and when these friendly bacteria die, the vaginal mucous membrane becomes susceptible to Candida invasion.

Feminine Hygiene Products
In the West we live in a super-hygienic deodorized society, and this is

reflected in every aspect of our lives. A woman's genital area has a natural odour, yet this seems to be considered unpleasant in some quarters. Advertising compounds our insecurities about ourselves by implying that we can only be really feminine if we use 'intimate feminine deodorants'. Absolute nonsense. I am not implying that we should not wash every day. Of course we should keep clean and fresh but we should not take this to excess. Feminine hygiene products are applied to extremely delicate tissues, which means that they are easily taken into the bloodstream and the toxic substances distributed throughout our bodies. Who knows what the effects are, but we do know that these products change the pH of the genital area, killing off acid-loving friendly bacteria and allowing the yeast to carve a little niche for itself.

Sexual Intercourse
Sexual intercourse also changes our pH. Many women complain that they develop thrush after sexual intercourse. Remember that the female genital tract is naturally acidic, as opposed to the alkaline pH of the male genital tract and the semen which men produce. A mingling of acid and alkaline brings the pH to neutral, which provides a less hospitable environment for the protective bacteria. The vigorous action of sexual intercourse can also erode the delicate tissues of the vagina. So we have a perfect situation in which Candida can proliferate and enter deeper tissue layers.

Hormone Therapy
The Pill and Hormone Replacement Therapy have revolutionized the lives of women. We can control when we become pregnant, and we can ease or even put off some of the unpleasant effects of the menopause. But what about the side-effects of these medications?

HRT and the Pill are made up of either synthesized hormones or the hormones derived from animal products such as mares' urine. Apart from the ethical issues that this may raise, these hormones are not natural to our bodies, and many women relate the onset of their Candida infection to the time when they started taking the Pill or HRT.

Environmental Hormones
Oestrogen hormones are everywhere. Farmers routinely include hormone treatment in animal feed to encourage faster growth and

greater milk production in their livestock. These hormones remain in the food which we eat, and are thus taken into our bodies. Even if you are a vegan and don't eat any of this food, you can still pick up environmental oestrogens in tap water, as some are excreted via the urine into our water systems. Urban water is recycled something like seven times (depending on where you live), and this is how you can inadvertently ingest environmental hormones into your body.

These environmental hormones are well known to exert an oestrogenic effect, and may even clog up your oestrogen hormone receptors, thus causing a relative progesterone dominance, or simply a hormonal imbalance.

What Can Be Done?

- Get tested for hormone imbalances.
- Avoid the Pill and HRT.
- Detoxify your body and focus on rebalancing your hormones.
- Eat organic foods.
- Reduce intake of meats, focus on vegetarian proteins instead.
- Stop using femine hygiene products.
- Douche with diluted lemon juice immediately after making love.
- If possible, avoid using antibiotics and steroid medications.
- Repopulate the vagina with probiotic pessaries.

If you think that a hormone imbalance might be contributing to your Candida problem, then ask your doctor or complementary medical practitioner to test your oestrogen and progesterone levels. If you are on the Pill, and want to come off, you are strongly advised to go to a family planning clinic where you will be advised of alternative methods of contraception.

If you are taking HRT, you have many alternative routes for the treatment of menopausal symptoms. Herbal medicine, nutritional medicine and homeopathy are only three of several options now available to women going through the menopause. Plant substances such as soya products, fennel seed, sage, black cohosh and red clover are a small example of the wide range of plant products that are abundant in phyto-oestrogens. These phyto-oestrogens (phyto = plant + oestrogens) are far more gentle on the body, and yet are superb in the treatment of menopausal symptoms. I have a woman patient who told me that when she first consulted me, she had been very sceptical that herbal medicine could possibly control her raging menopausal flushes and sweats. After only six weeks, however, her symptoms were under control. A list of professional bodies regulating various complementary therapies is supplied at the end of this book.

You can also try a gentle detox programme, using either dietary changes or herbal substances. This will allow oestrogen receptors to become unblocked, as well as giving your liver a break so that it can process all the toxins that will be released.

Try to focus on eliminating red meat from your diet. When you do eat meat, fish, eggs or dairy products, try to use organic products. These foods have far fewer contaminants such as antibiotics, hormones and pesticide residues. Try to concentrate on eating plenty of vegetables and salads, nuts and vegetable proteins.

Stop using feminine deodorants. You don't need them. If you find that thrush occurs after sexual intercourse, perhaps consider using a lubricant gel. Immediately after making love, have a bath and squeeze a lemon under the water between your legs to re-acidify the genital area.

To repopulate the vaginal bacteria, you can buy probiotic pessaries from a pharmacy or health food shop. Otherwise, you can make you own by dipping a tampon into plain live yoghurt and inserting it into your vagina for half an hour. To make this even more effective, you can open a probiotic capsule and mix it in with the yoghurt before applying to your vagina.

Treating hormone imbalances can be tricky. This book cannot in any way be a substitute for a professional consultation with a qualified complementary practitioner. You are strongly advised to consult a practitioner who will guide you through the process of regulating your hormones and detoxifying your body system, in a way that suits your individual needs.

Chapter Five

Blood Sugar and Your Diet

One of the major contributors to Candida is our modern diet, which is high in refined carbohydrates and sugars. Most people today eat as much as ten times the amount of sugar they would have eaten 100 years ago. Today people consider one chocolate bar a day to be a conservative intake of sugar! Our bodies are just not designed to deal with so much sugar. The 'Stone Age diet', which is the diet we humans are designed to live on, consists of whole grains, vegetables, fish, various meats and nuts, sugars derived from fruits and the occasional treat of honey.

The major impact that sugar has on our bodies with regard to Candida is that it feeds the sugar-hungry yeast, so it is necessary as part of any anti-Candida treatment programme to avoid sugars at all costs. Essentially, the anti-Candida diet focuses on avoiding sugars and yeasts. Many Candida sufferers become sensitized and allergic to yeast as a result of Candida invading beyond the confines of the intestine. Below you will find a brief list of the types of food that you should avoid, followed by an explanation as to why these foods should be avoided.

It is beyond the scope of this book to prescribe a full anti-Candida diet, but there are plenty of excellent books available on the market which do so. You will find that authors vary slightly in their approach. I would advise you to follow a strict rather than more lenient diet, as this way you will meet with greater success. Whichever diet you choose, you need to stick to it to see results.

You have probably heard horror stories about the restrictions of an anti-Candida diet. There is no doubt that it is probably one of the strictest diets that you will ever come across, but it does not need to be restrictive. In fact, it can be quite an exciting diet, because it forces you to look for alternatives to your normal diet. Many people have developed food sensitivities as a result of a leaky gut, and so alternatives to these foods must be found. This encourages you to explore foods from other cultures, and new ways of eating.

Sugars

Yeast loves sugar. Sugar is the Candida yeast's favourite food, and if you eat sugar, you are feeding your Candida, promoting its population explosion and your illness.

If you want to see what happens in your body when you eat sugar, try this little experiment:

- Fill two cups with warm water.
- Add a teaspoon of yeast to each and stir.
- Now add a teaspoon of sugar to just one of the cups and see what happens.
- Nothing will happen to the cup without the sugar, but in the sugary cup there will be a lot of activity. The yeast will soon start to bubble, froth and expand enormously.
- This is what happens to your body every time you eat sugar the yeast population expands, and also ferments the sugars, producing gas and alcohol.

During the first month of your anti-Candida diet, all sugars should be avoided. Even fruits should be avoided for the first month, after which you can start to include some fruit, but not the very sweet fruits like grapes or melons.

The usual advice is that all fruits should be avoided long term, but this is currently being debated. You will remember that in its fungal form, Candida relies on an oxygen-free environment to survive. The fruit sugar fructose is not metabolized in the same way as glucose, in that at a cellular level it actually *makes* oxygen, which helps to kill off the Candida.

There are great benefits to be derived from including the sweet-tasting powder FOS in your diet. FOS (fructo-oligo-saccharide) is derived from fructose, and feeds the friendly, beneficial bacteria, as well as aiding gut-wall healing. FOS is your loophole if you have a sweet tooth. It tastes like candy-floss and is actually good for you!

During the first month when you are avoiding fruits, you should make sure to supplement your vitamin and mineral intake by eating plenty of fresh vegetables, either raw or lightly steamed, and salads.

After the first month, if you go back to eating some fruits, start slowly by introducing the less sweet fruits such as apples and blueberries.

It is important to make sure that you don't feel hungry. When we feel hungry, our bodies scream for sugars to boost flagging blood sugar levels, and we start to crave sugary foods. Keep a stock of unsweetened oat biscuits, rice cakes or seeds with you so that you can regularly snack on these whenever you feel hungry.

Chromium polynicotinate, taken in a dose of 200 micrograms (mcg) per day, also helps to regulate blood sugar levels and thus prevent sugar cravings. Chromium is to be avoided, however, if you have diabetes and are using insulin.

Whatever you do avoid sugar. Keep this as your mantra: *By eating sugar, I am doing Candida a favour.*

Sugar-rich Foods
- all sugars
- honey
- syrups
- artificial sweeteners
- glucose, dextrose, fructose, sucrose
- jams (including sugar-free varieties)
- chocolates and sweets
- dried fruits
- diabetic sweets
- sweetened breakfast cereals
- fructose (in the first month) all fruits and fruit juices
- baked beans, tinned fruits and most tinned vegetables, which contain sugars
- canned soft drinks
- It is surprising how many hidden sugars there are in foods always read the label.

Refined Carbohydrates

Whole grains are an excellent source of vitamins and minerals, but food processing strips the goodness from the grain and leaves only the starch from which many of our foods are made. When carbohydrates are broken down in our digestive system, they are reduced to the components of which they are built – sugars. Refined carbohydrates are also very easily broken down, and so release the sugars quickly into our bloodstream, which of course feeds the yeast. This does not mean to say that you should avoid whole grains. These are good for you in that they provide fibre and nutrients. They also release their sugars slowly, and allow time for you to burn these sugars off as energy.

Foods Containing Refined Carbohydrates
- white flour
- white rice
- pasta
- cornflour
- custard powder
- baked beans
- refined breakfast cereals
- anything coated in breadcrumbs

Yeast Products
Because of the almost inevitable leaky gut which develops alongside Candida infection, the Candida yeast will escape into the bloodstream and your immune system will set up an antibody reaction to the yeast. As a result, your body will be intolerant of yeast and your immune system will need time to switch off this response. The only way to do this is to avoid completely any food or substance containing yeast or fungus for the first three months. This includes all fermented products. Certain smoked and cured processes also include yeast, so it is best to avoid these foods as well.

After this, you can experiment by eating some mushrooms and monitoring your reaction. If you feel a sudden onset of fogginess, bloating, headaches or sudden fatigue, you can be almost certain that you should avoid these foods for a longer period. Yeast and fungus is often hidden in foods, so once again, always read the label.

Foods Which Contain Yeast
- breads, buns, cakes, biscuits, pizza
- yeast spreads such as Marmite, Oxo, Bovril
- sauces such as Worcestershire sauce, tomato sauce (ketchup), barbecue sauces
- cheeses
- fungal foods such as mushrooms, truffles
- nuts (except those you crack yourself)
- smoked foods such as bacon, smoked fish

- vitamins made with a yeast base. Some are based on rice, and they are fine. Check the label and only buy if yeast-free.
- many antibiotics are based on moulds and yeasts
- the food additive monosodium glutamate, which is often derived from yeast

Fermented Products

Yeast is required to turn the sugar in fruit or grains into alcohol. If you are trying to avoid yeast, then it is imperative that you steer clear of fermented products. However, there is some disagreement about vinegar. In the past, experts used to advise that vinegar should be excluded from any anti-Candida diet. However, the National Candida Society notes that some research has found vinegar and vegetables pickled in vinegar are actually beneficial because they reduce the ability of the Candida to adhere to the gut wall. The Candida can then be more easily dislodged and removed via the bowel when you also include fibre-rich foods in your diet. Again, it is worth having a food intolerance test to check whether you are intolerant of vinegar and vinegar-rich products.

Fermented or Malted Products
- alcohol beer, wine, cider, spirits
- vinegar-containing products pickles, vinegar, ketchup, salad cream, baked beans, sauerkraut, horseradish-sauce
- soy sauce
- sourdough bread
- black tea

Smoked or Cured Products
- bacon
- smoked fish

Dairy Products

Cows' milk products are very unsuitable for an anti-Candida diet. As you have seen earlier, modern farming methods employ the regular use of antibiotics and hormone treatments, which find their way into the dairy produce. The antibiotics and hormones unbalance the hormonal and immune system, making you more vulnerable to Candida. Milk also contains a sugar known as lactose, which contributes to raising blood sugar levels and feeding the Candida yeast. Moreover, the fungus of mouldy cheeses will add a further load to your already exhausted immune system.

Cows' milk is made up of a very large protein called casein. This protein is not suitable for humans because we don't have the enzymes to digest it easily. Later on in the diet regime, you might include goats' or sheep's milk products, which have a much smaller protein molecule, and are consequently much more easily digested.

There are three dairy products where you will find a little leeway. Unsweetened, organic, plain live yoghurt can actually be of benefit by topping up levels of the friendly bacteria from which it is made. The protein molecule in this type of yoghurt is also partly digested by the friendly bacteria within the yoghurt, and is therefore much more acceptable to our digestive systems.

Butter is made primarily from the fat of the milk, and contains very little of the sugar and the protein which cause the trouble.

Cottage cheese is also fine to add to your diet once you have established that you are not intolerant or allergic to milk products.

I would suggest that these three products should be avoided for the first month of treatment, and then gradually introduced. Provided you have no allergies or food sensitivities to dairy products, you may include a small portion of each in your diet, but make sure that you use only organic and unsweetened cottage cheese and butter, and that the yoghurt is also 'live' or 'bioactive'.

Foods Containing Dairy Products
- ice-cream
- cream and fromage frais
- sweetened yoghurt
- milk, buttermilk
- cheese
- whey powder
- milk powder
- butter

Stimulants and Toxins
Stimulants do not directly raise blood sugar levels, but by stimulating the sympathetic nervous system, which induces the fight or flight response, blood sugar levels are raised so that the body is prepared for action. If physical action doesn't take place and burn off the

sugars, the yeast has a lovely feast of sugars to feed on.

Foods and Substances with a Stimulating Effect
- coffee
- tea
- cigarettes
- chocolate and hot chocolate drinks
- fizzy (carbonated) drinks
- guarana and other 'fat burners'

Tap Water
Tap water contains antibiotics, so use bottled spring water or purified water instead.

Toxins
A body infected with Candida already has a high toxic load due to the substances which have slipped through the leaky gut, so you should try to avoid putting even more toxins into your system by eliminating the following additives:
- monosodium glutamate
- food additives, preservatives, colours and flavourings
- sweeteners

Good News, Bad News

You have probably looked through the lists of foods you need to avoid in dismay, and decided that you are about to starve to death. Not true. You may feel that you can't possibly do without your morning coffee, toast and marmalade. The fact is that if you want to get better again, you have to. An anti-Candida diet is fundamental to curing your Candida problem. It simply doesn't make sense to try to heal the rest of your body and kill off the fungus while still providing it with its favourite food.

The good news is that the anti-Candida diet is an almost ideal diet. Through this diet you will be moving towards good health again, your hair and skin will improve, and you will lose weight without ever feeling hungry. This is not a calorie-restrictive diet, so eat as much as you want, but just make sure that you eat the right stuff. If you are concerned because you don't want to lose weight, then you can increase your calorific intake by eating plenty of nuts and seeds, which are high in fats. Proteins in the form of meat, oily fish and legumes will also contribute to keeping your weight up.

It is important that you eat a balanced diet and do not become malnourished on this diet. I would strongly advise that you consult a nutritionist to help you construct a balanced and nutritious diet. Your nutritionist will also assess your nutritional status and food sensitivities, and will prescribe supplements and a programme that suits your specific requirements.

Developing a Positive Attitude

Attitude counts a great deal. There is no doubt that it is very difficult to re-educate your palate after a lifetime of enjoying sweet foods. However, do try to focus on moving towards health rather than on suffering due to having to give up some of your favourites.

Sweet foods are often seen as a treat, so consider spending some time constructing a list of alternative treats for yourself so that you have something to refer to when you need to reward yourself. Perhaps a beautifully scented bath, or a facial treatment, a spa day out, maybe a new colour of nail polish or a new DVD, going ice-skating, seeing a movie, taking a boat trip or giving the dog a treat by walking him/her on a different route. Do anything – just avoid sugars at all costs!

You should bear in mind that you will need to stay off a high-sugar diet for the rest of your life. Your health is your choice; by following a healthy diet you are taking responsibility for your health. If you go back to eating a high-sugar diet your Candida will return, because you are feeding it.

How Long Must I Remain on This Diet?

This is probably the most commonly asked question, and also the most difficult to answer definitively. Initially you will need to be extremely strict, and exclude all sugars for six months, until the Candida is under control. After that you will be able to start to allow some leniency into the diet, but you need to understand that you will never be able to go back to a high-sugar, refined carbohydrate diet again. The good news is that after being sugar-free for so long, you will probably find you have lost your taste for over-sweet foods and drinks.

It is not always necessary to avoid yeast products for ever. If you have become sensitized to yeast, then you will need to avoid yeast for at least six months, but if you are not sensitive to yeast, then there is no reason why it should not be included in your diet. You can check if you are sensitive to yeast by undergoing a food-sensitivity test (see Chapter Nine for further details.)

A Short List of Foods You Can Eat
Provided you have no allergic or intolerant reactions to these foods, you can include as many and as much of them as you like.

Carbohydrates
- Yeast-free organic breads: wholewheat soda bread, Rosinski, Borodinski, unleavened bread, unmalted oatcakes, rice cakes, Ryvita, sesame crispbreads
- Potatoes and sweet potatoes
- Wholewheat pasta
- Fibre-rich foods, especially linseeds or psyllium seeds.
- Home-made muesli, with nuts and seeds
- Grains: millet, brown rice, quinoa, spelt, oats

Proteins
- Organic meat and poultry
- Deep-sea fish and organic fresh-water fish
- Free-range organic eggs
- Beans and pulses preferably ones you cook yourself from raw, but tinned (unsweetened) are fine
- Cottage cheese
- Live, plain, organic yoghurt
- Seeds and nuts (with shells you crack yourself)

Fats
- Butter
- Unhydrogenated margarines especially olive oil-based margarines
- Olive oil

Vegetables and Fruits
- Fruits: Avocado pears, coconuts, lemons, tomatoes (after the first

month, include pineapples, kiwi, pawpaw and the berry fruits. Make sure you alternate your fruits daily)
- Onions, leeks and garlic
- Fresh vegetables and salads especially raw or juiced
- All herbs – especially oregano and thyme, which are anti-fungal

Alternatives to Dairy Products
- Soya milk, oat milk, rice milk, almond milk
- Rice and soya 'cheese' slices
- Soya-based 'cheese' spreads

Sweet Substitutes and Snacks
- Popcorn
- Hummus and tzatziki on crispbreads
- Vanilla essence and cinnamon provide sweet tastes without the sugar
- Cashew nuts and coconuts
- FOS

Beverages
- Rooibosch tea
- Pau D'Arco tea (anti-fungal)
- Chamomile tea
- Barleycup
- Dandelion coffee
- Home-made iced ginger/lemon/lemon balm/mint tea

This list is by no means comprehensive. I strongly advise that you purchase one of the excellent anti-Candida recipe books available on the market for a wider range of options and delicious recipes.

Chapter Six

Mercury Amalgam Dental Fillings

If you have Candida, but have not used therapeutic drugs that may have made you vulnerable to a fungal overgrowth, do not have a high-sugar diet, hormonal imbalance or an impaired immune system, it is possible that mercury dental fillings could be your problem.

Mercury is an extremely toxic substance, and links have been found between mercury toxicity and recurrent fungal disease, immune and hormonal disturbances and, significantly, kidney disease. It has also been suggested that mercury is probably implicated in Alzheimer's disease, multiple sclerosis and autism.

Mercury fillings (or 'silver stars' as they were called by the smiling dentist with a drill in his hand, when we were children) contain between 46 and 56 per cent metallic mercury, which is constantly released as mercury vapour into the body for many years after placement. The release of the mercury vapour is made worse by the ingestion of hot foods, chewing, food acids, and exposure to oxygen in the breath. The result is that those who have mercury amalgams are exposed to vastly elevated levels of mercury toxicity, which has a very detrimental effect on the body.

One of the earliest signs of mercury poisoning is forgetfulness, which may progress to an inability to concentrate, irritability and depression, fatigue, headaches and mood swings. Other signs may be poor co-ordination, numbness and tingling of the lips and the hands and feet, muscular weakness, impaired vision, kidney damage and immune dysfunction, among others. Later in the book you will notice how many signs of mercury poisoning are identical to the symptoms of Candida infection.

Of particular interest to Candida sufferers is the effect that mercury can have on the hormonal system, the immune system and the bacterial populations of the body.

Scientists as far back as 1971 noted that women exposed to mercury experienced painful and heavy menstrual bleeding, disturbances in their menstrual cycle and pre-menstrual tension. Other studies show a correlation between mercury exposure, spontaneous abortion and decreased fertility among women. One test showed that women experiencing difficulty conceiving had a 70 per cent success rate of becoming pregnant once their mercury fillings were removed. Male fertility is also affected by mercury, which is associated with impaired sperm motility.

Another very common sign of mercury poisoning affecting the hormonal system is abnormal hair growth in different parts of the body, or abnormal hair loss. While fertility may not be directly affected by or associated with Candida infection, these studies do indicate the significant detrimental effect that mercury can have on our hormones.

A study measuring the total percentages of T-cells in the blood showed that mercury is associated with a significant drop in T-cells and immune function. After the removal of mercury dental fillings, the T-cell population rose on average by a significant 43 per cent.

To further compound the problem, mercury has the effect of making intestinal bacteria resistant to oral antibiotics. Now, this might seem like a good thing, but unfortunately it is not. Remember that within our gut live both beneficial and non-beneficial bacteria. Should the balance between the two become compromised, and the non-beneficial bacteria begin to dominate, we will become ill. With an impaired immune system due to mercury poisoning, we are less likely to be able to ward off the infection by ourselves, and so it might become necessary to use antibiotics. Now, if these bad bacteria are resistant to the antibiotics, and we don't get better, it stands to reason that the doctor who is taking care of you will go on to prescribe a different course of antibiotics, and so on. In the mean time, our poor friendly bacteria are taking a real battering and the Candida will thrive.

If you believe that mercury dental fillings may be contributing to your Candida problem, please contact a dentist who is sympathetic to the idea of replacing these fillings for you.

Chapter Seven

The Ravaging Fungus

Once the Candida yeast has been allowed to change into its invasive fungal form, its root-like mycelia allow the Candida to penetrate into the interior of the body where its effects on the host's mental and physical well-being can be devastating.

The symptoms of Candida are so wide-ranging that they may seem to be totally unconnected. The following case study will give you an idea of how diverse the symptoms of Candida can be.

Susan first came to see me because she felt physically and mentally very tired all the time. She had had numerous blood tests through her general practitioner and other specialists, but the doctors could find nothing in the test results to point to the cause of her malaise.

After close questioning, Susan reported that she was experiencing bloating and excess gas in her stomach, and felt especially tired and nauseous after eating certain foods. Further questioning revealed that she almost always felt achy in her muscles and joints, suffered frequent headaches, and found it very difficult to concentrate, often having a feeling of mental fogginess. She ruefully laughed and commented on what a wreck she was, but after a treatment programme for Candida, her symptoms started to abate.

Candida has such a wide range of possible symptoms that the list below is only an example of the more common ones.
- abdominal bloating and gas
- leaky gut and food intolerance
- itchy anus
- thick white coating in the mouth, vagina and/or anus
- constant sugar cravings
- diarrhoea or constipation
- thrush
- cystitis
- loss of libido

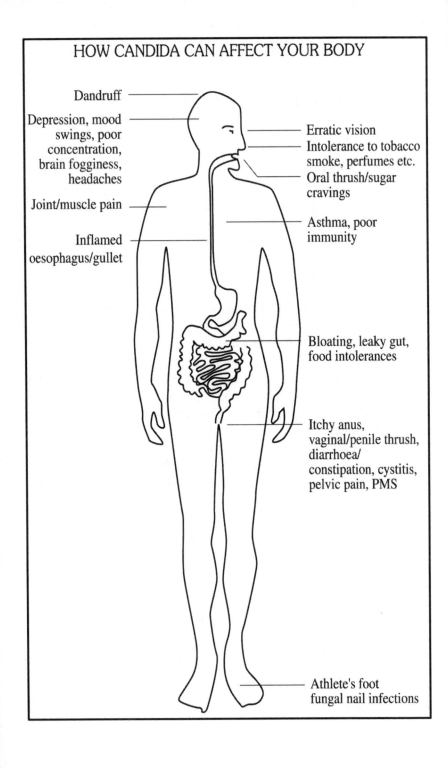

HOW CANDIDA CAN AFFECT YOUR BODY

Dandruff

Depression, mood swings, poor concentration, brain fogginess, headaches

Joint/muscle pain

Inflamed oesophagus/gullet

Erratic vision

Intolerance to tobacco smoke, perfumes etc.

Oral thrush/sugar cravings

Asthma, poor immunity

Bloating, leaky gut, food intolerances

Itchy anus, vaginal/penile thrush, diarrhoea/ constipation, cystitis, pelvic pain, PMS

Athlete's foot fungal nail infections

- excessive pre-menstrual symptoms● nagging pelvic pain
- athlete's foot
- fungal nail infections
- skin rashes
- dandruff
- asthma and hayfever
- excessive nasal catarrh
- joint and muscle pain
- pain behind the breastbone
- constant tiredness and lethargy
- depression
- brain fogginess and poor concentration
- mood swings
- frequent headaches
- erratic vision
- intolerance of perfumes and other smells
- poor immunity

Let us now examine how some of the effects of Candida occur in various parts of the body, and what can be done to claim back health.

The Digestive System

Some of the Candida symptoms associated with the digestive system include bloating and excess gas in the abdomen, sugar cravings, food sensitivities, and thrush in the mouth, oesophagus and around the anus.

Remember what happens when you use yeast to raise bread? Sugars are the catalyst which starts the fermentation process. There is a great production of gas, and an enormous expansion of the yeast cell population. This is exactly what happens in your digestive system when Candida overgrowth occurs. Satisfied sugar cravings feed the yeast population, which is allowed to expand far beyond healthy proportions if the friendly bacterial population and immune system are compromised. When the yeast grows, it produces lots of fermentation gasses, which are translated into the symptoms of excess gas, bloating and abdominal discomfort.

Under these conditions, the Candida yeast changes into its fungal form and the root-like mycelia penetrate the gut wall, producing a porous, 'leaky' gut. The mucous membrane of the gut is so inflamed and damaged that it is neither able to secrete the correct amount of digestive acids and enzymes which break down food into smaller molecules, nor to absorb these essential nutritional molecules properly. The body is malnourished and, without this essential source of fuel, becomes exhausted.

The porous gut lining allows undigested food particles, chemical toxins and Candida fragments to escape from the confines of the digestive tract into the bloodstream and the interior environment of the body. The liver is the detoxification organ of the body, and the toxins which escape into the interior of the body, as well as the toxins secreted by the Candida, can lead to a toxic overload on the liver. This results in the host frequently developing sensitivities to chemicals such as perfumes, as well as feelings of nausea and sluggishness. Skin rashes, headaches and muscle pain can also be the result of toxic overload.

The alert immune system immediately sets up antibody reactions against these invaders. As a result, the body becomes sensitized to certain foods. The more food allergies develop, the more depleted your immune system becomes, and the less able it is to defend against the Candida invasion.

By now, the Candida is definitely gaining the upper hand, and is able to invade almost every part of the body. The thrush, which is apparent in the mouth and anus, indicates how Candida can spread through the digestive tract literally from mouth to anus. As the Candida invades the mucous membranes of the body, it causes inflammation, and the pain that many sufferers feel behind their breastbone indicates the inflammatory process occurring in the oesophagus, which is situated directly behind the breastbone.

So we have a body which is severely compromised by an increased toxic load, an overworked and depleted immune system, and insufficient nutrients to support the healing process. No wonder you feel exhausted.

The Immune System

You already know that the potential for Candida to become invasive is greater if the immune system is under stress, but Candida can actually directly attack and suppress the immune system, through various mechanisms.

When the Candida changes from the innocuous yeast form into its fungal form, it releases substances that cause inflammation to the gut wall, and then penetrates the gut-lining barrier with root-like mycelia. This damages the mucous membrane as well as the numerous immune tissues that line the wall. The damage to the gut wall's immune-defence mechanism allows other, previously controlled organisms such as bacteria, viruses or protozoa to enter the bloodstream and make further demands on the already stressed immune system.

Invading foreign organisms, undigested food particles and chemical toxins are referred to as *antigens*, and are all subjected to antibody attack. The antibodies and antigens combine to form 'antigen antibody immune complexes', which may be stored at various sites in the body. Immune complexes stored in the lungs lead to symptoms such as asthma; those stored in the joints and muscles cause symptoms such as hot, swollen, painful joints and muscles; complexes deposited in the brain tissue may result in what are known as brain allergies. Candida itself is also made up of at least 79 substances which can produce an allergic immune response in the body. The production of antibodies places great demands on the humoral immune resources.

Some of the invading antigens so closely resemble our own tissue cells that the immune system may confuse the antigen with 'self-tissue', and eventually start to attack our own tissues. This leads to what are known as 'auto-immune diseases', and scientists have supported this by demonstrating that Candida can directly cross-react with human tissue, and result in the development of auto-immune disease.

Candida can also play a direct role in suppressing cellular immunity through the release of toxins, of which nearly 100 have been isolated thus far. Toxins such as acetyldehyde and carbon monoxide act specifically to suppress the T-cell arm of the cellular immune system. This is a very clever move by Candida, as cellular immunity is the part of the immune system that directly attacks the Candida fungus.

You can see how devastating Candida can be to the body's defence system: through the production of multiple antigens, Candida imposes on the B-cell (humoral) arm of the immune system, and directly suppresses the T-cell mediated arm of the immune system.

Apart from Candida taking advantage of a weak immune system to invade the body, it potentially has a powerful and devastating effect of its own on the immune system:

- Damage to the gut wall destroys the immune tissues situated within the mucous membrane.
- Foreign invading antigens provoke an antibody response by the immune system, which further depletes resources.
- Candida produces at least 79 of its own antigens to further challenge the immune system.
- These antigens have a documented potential to cause auto-immune disease in sufferers of systemic Candida.
- Candida produces toxins which directly suppress the T-cell arm of the immune system.
- Candida fungus imposes on, or directly suppresses, both arms of the white blood cell immune system of its host.

The Nervous System

It is not perfectly well understood exactly how Candida affects the nervous system, but there are several theories. One theory focuses on the undigested protein particles, which gain entry into the bloodstream via the leaky gut. These protein molecules may have endorphin-like actions, which can influence our moods. Endorphins are substances produced by the brain which have powerful pain-relieving properties, and influence our mood, behaviour, memory and sexual activity. The undigested proteins which slip in through the leaky gut originate from outside of the body, are not natural to the body, and therefore have been termed *exorphins*. Exorphins slot into the receptors in the brain and can affect the mood of the Candida sufferer by turning on or off neurological reactions as if they were pushing buttons.

Another theory again centres on the undigested proteins which enter the bloodstream and encounter the B-cells of the immune system. As mentioned, the B-cells secrete antibodies which combine with the protein antigen to form antigen-antibody immune complexes. These complexes are deposited at various sites in the body, including the brain, joints, kidneys and lungs. The complexes deposited in the brain set up a 'brain allergy' response and cause the host to suffer from depression, mood swings, memory problems and poor co-ordination. Although brain allergies may not be directly related to Candida, it is clear that Candida can cause this response because of its action of damaging the gut wall. Note the astounding similarity between the neurological symptoms of Candida and the neurological symptoms of an allergy. Clearly the two mechanisms are linked.

Neurological Symptoms of Candida
- depression
- frequent headaches
- lethargy and fatigue
- brain fogginess
- mood swings
- poor memory
- poor concentration
- loss of libido
- autism
- fungal meningitis

Neurological Symptoms of Allergy
- emotional instability
- headaches
- fatigue
- indecisiveness
- impaired co-ordination
- disorientation
- poor memory
- loss of libido

Candida can affect the body through various mechanisms. Above we saw that the fungus can have a powerful influence over the nervous system as a result of the damage caused to the gut wall. However, it is clear that Candida exerts its effects through more than one method.

Japanese studies have shown that the toxins produced by Candida can have severe effects on the nervous system, leading to conditions such as depression, schizophrenia and even autism.

A healthy little boy with the usual interest in and alertness to his family and surroundings developed a series of ear infections, and was given several courses of antibiotics by his family doctor. Soon after this, the boy's speech development stopped. He then became unresponsive and withdrawn, and eventually progressed to muteness. A few months later he was diagnosed with late-onset autism.

Could this be a very severe attack of Candida? Dr Bernard Rimland of the Autism Research Institute, San Diego, believes that this particular boy did indeed suffer from a severe attack of Candida which left his immune system in tatters. The boy was treated for Candida and he is now once again a lively and happy fellow. Dr Rimland and other experts in the field of Candida believe that 5 to 15 per cent of autistic children would improve if they were treated for Candida.

The Hormonal System

Candida has been implicated in several conditions which are caused by hormone imbalances, such as pre-menstrual syndrome and endometriosis. Candida has a steroid-binding protein, and as hormones are derived from steroids, this means Candida is capable of binding with progesterone and other hormones of the endocrine (hormonal) system. Once Candida is bound to the hormone, it is capable of participating in or interfering with hormonal signals.

Pre-menstrual Syndrome
Pre-menstrual syndrome is caused by an imbalance of progesterone, although a general hormonal imbalance has been suggested. The ability of Candida to bind to progesterone means that available progesterone levels may be reduced sufficiently to predispose a woman to the development of pre-menstrual syndrome.

Endometriosis
Although the exact cause of endometriosis is still unknown, there is a strong correlation between a Candida overgrowth and the development of endometriosis. It has been suggested that the mycelia of the Candida fungus are capable of penetrating the wall of the uterus (womb), as with the gut wall, and this allows pieces of uterine tissue to escape into the body, where they attach to inappropriate sites and continue to respond to hormonal influences, by bleeding every month during menstruation. The bleeding causes scar tissue to develop inside the abdominal cavity, and this scar tissue acts as ropes adhering to many internal structures, pulling with each move-

ment and causing great discomfort and pain to the sufferer.

Auto-immune Hormonal Conditions

It appears that the immune system becomes confused by the steroid-binding protein of the yeast, and arranges an immune response against the steroids and hormones of the endocrine system. In doing so, the immune system begins to attack its own endocrine tissues, thus setting the scene for the development of auto-immune disease. This phenomenon was first described by the late Phyllis Saider, an endocrinologist who in the mid-1980s termed this event 'APICH syndrome' (APICH stands for Auto-immune Polyendocrinopathy Immune-dysregulation Candidosis Hypersensitivity).

APICH Syndrome

APICH syndrome may be identified as an auto-immune endocrine disorder affecting all sufferers of Candida who just don't seem to get better, despite the correct treatment. The thyroid gland, adrenal glands and ovaries are the major glands involved, although others such as the pancreas may also be affected. The most common symptoms of this syndrome include overwhelming fatigue, depression and short-term memory loss, but patients with APICH syndrome are also prone to developing the auto-immune conditions and related symptoms described in the list below.

- thyroiditis and hypothyroidism – physical and mental fatigue, sensitivity to cold, dry hair and skin
- oophoritis – painful inflammation of the ovaries
- hypoadrenalism and Addison's disease – depression, weakness and fatigue, skin pigmentation, dizziness, nausea and weight loss
- diabetes mellitus – a disease affecting the pancreas where the body is unable to control blood sugar levels
- pre-menstrual syndrome

Other disorders related to APICH syndrome include:

- hypo-parathyroidism - a condition where the parathyroid glands do not secrete enough of their calcium regulating hormones, and this results in abnormally low levels of calcium in the blood
- pernicious anaemia

- hepatitis
- alopecia
- vitiligo
- myasthenia gravis - a serious disorder where there is exceptional muscular weakness caused by antibodies preventing the nerve impulses from signaling to the muscles to contract
- pemphigus - an uncommon skin disorder which is caused by the bodies antibodies causing damage to the skin, and resulting in large blisters, which burst and leave the underlying skin raw and crusting.
- allergic rhinitis hay fever
- schizophrenia
- autism
- sprue - a disease which occurs mainly in the tropics, and characterised by diarrhoea with fat globules in the stool, anaemia, a sore tongue and weight loss)
- coeliac disease
- testiculitis
- pituitary deficiency
- systemic lupus erythematosis - an autoimmune condition found mainly in women, and characterized by red skin on the face, aching joints, hair loss and other internal organ damage.
- rheumatoid arthritis
- Sjogren's syndrome – a dryness of the mouth and eyes, often combined with rheumatoid arthritis
- Goodpasture's syndrome - a serious disease where the antibodies attack the lungs and kidney tissues resulting in coughing blood and kidney failure

The APICH syndrome is described in: Trowbridge & Walker (1986) The Yeast Syndrome, Bantam Books. The authors cite the proceedings of the 1985 Yeast-Human Interaction Symposium.

When considering the effects of Candida albicans on the human body, we seem to have a scale, with a mild bout of thrush at one end and APICH syndrome at the other, severe end of the scale. Wherever your experience of Candida lies, it is absolutely imperative that you bear in mind that this is a condition of an unbalanced environment, and it is that which you need to treat. You cannot simply kill off the fungus and expect that your problem will go away.

Summary of the Causes of a Candida Overgrowth

Poor immunity, caused by the following:
- stress
- poor nutrition
- immune-suppressive diseases such as HIV, Chronic Fatigue Syndrome
- immuno-suppressive drug therapy for organ transplants and auto-immune diseases
- chemotherapy for cancer treatment
- long-term or recurrent steroid therapy
- long-term or repeated antibiotic therapy
- environmental antibiotics found in meat, fish, eggs and dairy products

High blood sugar levels, caused by the following:
- a diet high in sugars and refined carbohydrates
- stress
- stimulants such as coffee
- diseases such as diabetes and Syndrome X

Hormonal imbalances, which may be caused by the following:
- hormone therapy Hormone Replacement Therapy, the Pill, natural progesterone cream
- hormonal changes puberty, pre-menstrual phase of the monthly cycle, pregnancy, menopause
- steroid therapy treatment for asthma, eczema, arthritis and other inflammatory diseases
- environmental hormones steroids found in food products, and oestrogen in the water supply

Changes in pH balance, which may be caused by the following:
- the use of feminine hygiene products
- sexual intercourse

Chapter Eight

Candida and Traditional Chinese Medicine

Now comes a very interesting twist in the tale. In Traditional Chinese Medicine, Candida may be referred to as a disease of 'Dampness'. Traditional Chinese Medicine (TCM) is an extremely complex medical system, so please understand that this is just a simplified outline of the association between Eastern and Western approaches to Candida.

According to the principles of TCM, 'Dampness' is heavy and interferes with the Yang (the hot, exuberant 'male' energy, which normally is balanced by the cool, deep 'female' (Yin) energy within each of us) of the body. Damp also impedes the transformational function of food and liquids into Qi (energy) by the spleen. As well as interfering with spleen function, Dampness may also be caused by a weakness of the Spleen (digestion).

By interfering with balance in the body, Damp may manifest with a feeling of heaviness and lethargy, bloating, a general loss of energy and associated mental confusion. There may be stiffness and swelling in the joints, a fever, a thick tongue coating, a thick vaginal discharge and thin, brittle hair. All of these symptoms are made worse by humid conditions.

Dampness is believed to be a result of weakness in the Spleen. The spleen (analogous to the digestive system in Western medicine) is responsible for the transformation of foods and liquids into Qi. If this function is disrupted, the result is Dampness and Phlegm, which is an advanced form of Damp. Damp may also be caused by disharmony in the Kidneys, which are involved in governing water in the body, or by the lungs, which control the dispersion of defensive Qi (immune function) and body fluids throughout the body.

Note the similarities between the Eastern and Western understanding of Candida:
- Dampness may be caused by a weakness of the Spleen, which is analogous to the digestive system in Western anatomy. This is the

region of the body where the Candida yeast may change into its fungal form.

- Damp may also be caused by a weakness of the Lungs, which disperse the Defensive Qi and whose function is analogous to the immune defence system.
- Both conditions are worse in humid conditions.
- Dampness and Candida have similar symptoms.

Comparison Between the Symptoms and Treatment of Candida and 'Dampness'

Candida	Dampness
Lethargy and fatigue	Heaviness and lethargy
Abdominal bloating	Abdominal bloating
Mental confusion	Mental confusion
Pain in the muscles and joints	Pain and swelling in the joints
Poor control of body temperature	Possibly a fever or a chill
Oral thrush	Thick tongue coating
Vaginal thrush	Thick vaginal discharges
Food intolerances with catarrh	Mucus or phlegm in the chest or stool
Treatment involves avoiding sugars, refined carbohydrates	Avoidance of sweet, greasy or stodgy foods
Using anti-fungal herbs and spices such as cinnamon, ginger	Use of hot dispersing herbs and and spices such as cinnamon, cloves, ginger, thyme, oregano, savory, juniper, lemons

If you prefer to treat your Candida from a Traditional Chinese Medical perspective, then you might consider consulting a good acupuncturist, or even better, an acupuncturist who is also a practising Chinese Herbalist.

Part Two

Chapter Nine

Diagnosing Candida

It is really very difficult to make a *completely definitive* decision as to whether a person has Candida or not. In the past, practitioners could only hazard an educated guess by taking a very good case history and, based on the patient's clinical picture, design a treatment programme for Candida. If the patient responded to the treatment, then the practitioner congratulated him- or herself on the correct diagnosis, and the patient recovered. These days, we are lucky enough to have non-invasive tests which can give an accurate assessment of whether or not someone has a disorder related to *Candida albicans*.

There are a variety of tests which are appropriate for Candida, but a good case history, as always, is the most valuable. A practitioner familiar with Candida should be able to make a fairly accurate diagnosis, and then confirm the diagnosis with the most appropriate tests for your particular condition.

A Self-scoring Diagnostic Test

Tick the boxes in this simple self-scoring diagnostic test. If you tick at least one in Box A, and six or more in Box B, then you have a strong reason to believe that you may have yeast-related health problems.

Please bear in mind that while this questionnaire is useful to suggest whether or not you have Candida, it is simply not accurate enough, as Candida has so many symptoms which overlap with other disease conditions. It is very important that other diseases are ruled out before commencing with treatment for Candida. For this reason you are strongly advised to consult a practitioner who can guide you towards the most appropriate tests for an accurate diagnosis.

A. Causes of Candida

Have you taken the following medicines?
- ☐ antibiotics for eight weeks or more?
- ☐ antibiotics for short periods four or more times in a year?
- ☐ steroids for asthma, eczema, arthritis, any other reason?
- ☐ the contraceptive pill for a year or more?
- ☐ Hormone Replacement Therapy for a year or more?
- ☐ immuno-suppressive drugs?

Do you suffer from the following conditions?
- ☐ Diabetes mellitus
- ☐ Chronic Fatigue Syndrome (ME)
- ☐ recurrent bacterial or viral infections
- ☐ AIDS or HIV

- ☐ Have you had multiple pregnancies?

B. Symptoms of Candida
Hormonal Symptoms

Do you regularly experience the following symptoms?
- ☐ recurrent oral or vaginal thrush
- ☐ vaginitis (inflammation, redness and soreness of the vagina)
- ☐ a loss of libido
- ☐ recurrent cystitis or urinary tract infections
- ☐ pre-menstrual syndrome, or menstrual irregularities
- ☐ a flare-up of thrush symptoms prior to your period
- ☐ a flare-up of thrush symptoms immediately after sexual intercourse
- ☐ Have you experienced an unaccountable weight loss or gain without a change of diet?
- ☐ Do you suffer from endometriosis?

Intestinal Symptoms
Do you suffer from the following symptoms?
- ☐ abdominal bloating
- ☐ diarrhoea or constipation
- ☐ itchy anus
- ☐ food allergies or intolerance

- [ ] sugar cravings
- [ ] bad breath
- [ ] belching or flatulence
- [ ] difficulty swallowing
- [ ] indigestion or heartburn
- [ ] mucus in stools

Neurological Symptoms
Are the following symptoms present?
- [ ] mood swings or depression
- [ ] fatigue and lethargy
- [ ] poor concentration and poor memory
- [ ] foggy brain
- [ ] poor co-ordination
- [ ] loss of balance
- [ ] headaches and migraines
- [ ] Does exposure to strong smells such as tobacco, perfumes or other fumes affect you?
- [ ] Do you experience erratic vision?

Other Symptoms
Are the following symptoms present?
- [ ] athlete's foot or any other fungal skin or nail infections
- [ ] persistent dandruff
- [ ] muscle or joint aches
- [ ] unaccountable skin rashes
- [ ] nasal congestion, hay fever or fluid in the ear
- [ ] pain behind the breast bone

Are your symptoms worse in the following conditions?
- [ ] on damp days, or in a damp climate
- [ ] when exposed to mouldy vegetation matter
- [ ] in a mouldy house
- [ ] near a foggy beach

Diagnostic Tests Available

Gut Fermentation Test

This test measures the level of alcohol in the blood before and after the ingestion of sugar. If alcohol appears in the blood after the ingestion of sugar, this suggests that fermentation is taking place. However, this test is unable to identify clearly what is causing the fermentation to occur, as there is evidence pointing towards the fact that bacteria, as well as yeast, can ferment sugar.

Candida Stool Culture Test

This is one of the older tests used to diagnose Candida. The test requires a stool sample, and uses a special culture medium and the correct reduced oxygen conditions to grow and identify Candida. The disadvantage of this test is that, as *Candida albicans* is normally present in the gut, the presence of it in the stool cannot be used to diagnose an overgrowth of *Candida albicans* accurately. The strong advantage of this test is that it can be used to identify different species of Candida which should not normally be present in the body.

Candida Urine Test

This test looks for the presence of Candida in the urine. Candida would only be present in the urine if it had caused a local infection such as thrush or a urinary tract infection. So, while this test is valid for the diagnosis of a local infection, it cannot detect systemic Candida infection.

Blood or Saliva ELISA Test

When Candida yeast changes into its fungal form, it penetrates the gut wall and enters the bloodstream where it encounters the immune system, which releases antibodies specific to Candida. The ELISA test measures for these specific antibodies in the blood or saliva, and is able to assess accurately whether there is a systemic infection of Candida or not. The test is further refined by measuring immunoglobulin G, the presence of which indicates a long-term or old infection, and immunoglobulin A, which would suggest a more recent or active infection.

The great advantages of this test are that it is non-invasive (in that a saliva sample is as effective as a blood sample) and it is extremely accurate at determining whether there is a systemic infection of Candida or not.

One disadvantage is that the ELISA test measures only *Candida albicans*. As previously mentioned, there are approximately 400 species of Candida thus far identified. Even though 90 per cent of Candida-related problems are caused by *Candida albicans*, in a small number of cases the results could come back negative if the person is suffering from a yeast infection caused by a different species of Candida.

Another disadvantage of this test is that, in a very small number of cases, the immune system may be so deficient (due to Candida infection) that there are too few immunoglobulins to give a positive result, and so, ironically, the test result is a false negative, when in fact the person is very ill due to Candida.

Despite these two disadvantages, at the present time this does seem to be the most reliable means of testing for *Candida albicans* infection.

Other Appropriate Tests
Thyroid Function
One of the endocrine glands most commonly affected by Candida is the thyroid gland.

Symptoms of an under active thyroid include fatigue, weight gain concurrent with no change of diet, sensitivity to cold, dry scaly skin and hair, depression and poor concentration. An overactive thyroid may manifest with irritability and anxiety, feeling of heat, palpitations, weight loss without a change of diet and change of menstrual pattern. As many of these symptoms overlap with those of Candida, you would be strongly advised to consider this test.

Adrenal Stress Index
Chronic stress, long-term anti-inflammatory medication and a systemic Candida infection can adversely affect the adrenal glands, leading to symptoms such as weakness, fatigue, dizziness, sensitivity to cold, nausea and skin pigmentation. This test is advisable in order to assess whether the adrenal glands need attention.

Oestrogen/Progesterone Profile
Adult females are far more prone to developing Candida than other

members of the population, and women tend to become particularly susceptible immediately prior to their period. As discussed earlier in this book, thus far it has been impossible to prove one way or another whether it is oestrogen or progesterone which is to blame, but what is certainly apparent is that Candida is strongly associated with a hormonal imbalance. If you are a woman, it is vital that you have your female hormone levels checked.

Blood Glucose Levels

Fungus thrives in a sugar-rich environment. Sufferers of diabetes are particularly prone to developing Candida or fungal infections. If you have no other reason for suspecting why you should have developed Candida, do consider your blood glucose levels. Symptoms of diabetes include great thirst and increased urine output, skin and nail fungal infections, thrush, sudden mood swings and weight loss, even with an increased dietary intake. Diabetes is a serious disorder with several symptoms similar to those of Candida, and it needs to be treated by a medical practitioner urgently.

Food Intolerance/Allergy Test

Food allergies are strongly associated with Candida, and often it is your favourite foods to which you may have developed a sensitivity. Once these foods are eliminated or restricted in your diet, you will have taken a great step towards wellness.

Vitamin and Mineral Screen

Candida damages the gut membrane, and this severely compromises the ability of this membrane to absorb nutrients. Almost invariably, all Candida sufferers are deficient in certain vitamins and minerals, which further contributes towards illness. It is important to have your vitamin and mineral status assessed, so that any deficiencies may be corrected.

Diagnostic Outline

1. Complete the self-scoring questionnaire.
2. Get tested for *Candida albicans*.
3. Other appropriate tests include:
   - thyroid function

- cortisol levels / Adrenal Stress Index
- oestrogen/progesterone profile
- blood glucose levels
- food allergy or intolerance test
- vitamin and mineral screen

Chapter Ten

A Treatment Programme

In order to treat a condition effectively it is imperative that you understand the nature of what you are treating. Armed with the information provided in this book, you will understand that treating Candida effectively *cannot* involve merely 'killing off the fungus'. Although treatment does kill the fungus, it primarily involves rebalancing the internal environment so that the fungus cannot take hold again. If you only use anti-fungal medications without addressing the deeper underlying cause of the illness, as soon as the course of medication is finished the fungus population will simply explode again. Worse than that, those fungal organisms which survived the medication will reproduce a strain that is resistant to medication, so your problem will become worse than ever and even more embedded. However, if you focus on making the environment inhospitable to Candida, it won't be able to survive anywhere apart from where it belongs as a small population within your digestive system.

Candida infection is a complicated disorder. The treatment programme, while not complicated, is certainly complex. Once again, I would like to point out that this book should serve only as a guide and can never replace the expertise of a trained and qualified practitioner. By consulting a practitioner you will know that you have been correctly diagnosed and are supported in your treatment programme.

This treatment programme is designed to be used as a single unit. It is unlikely that you will get better if you focus on only one or other aspect of it. The programme may sound difficult, but once you get used to it you'll find it is not. Below is an outline of the treatment programme. Later in this chapter you will find much more detail relating to each point.

The Ten-Point Candida Treatment Programme

1. Get the correct diagnosis.

2. Follow the anti-Candida diet.

3. Take anti-fungal medications.

4. Heal the leaky gut wall.

5. Repopulate the intestine with probiotics.

6. Aid the digestive process.

7. Support the liver.

8. Rebalance the hormones.

9. Treat the immune system.

10. Redress your lifestyle.

Getting the Correct Diagnosis

You have seen that Candida can appear with many symptoms, several of which overlap with those of other disorders. For this reason it is very important that other diseases are ruled out before commencing with a treatment strategy for Candida. Make sure that it is Candida that is your problem by consulting a qualified practitioner.

Removing the Cause of Overgrowth

Before even starting the treatment programme, it is important that you evaluate and remove or redress the causes of the Candida overgrowth. If it is medication that started the Candida overgrowth, discuss this with your doctor and ask if you can change your medication. In some cases, such as the Pill, your doctor can suggest an alternative. If your doctor has no alternative to offer you, then it may be worth trying a complementary medical approach to address why it is that you need to be on this medication in the first place.

There are times when it is simply not possible to stop medication, but there are many cases when an alternative approach can treat both the Candida and the original, underlying problem. If it is your diet and lifestyle, try to change these by following the anti-Candida diet and finding ways to alleviate stress such as yoga, meditation, counselling or even boxing!

The disorders which Candida itself may have caused for you also need to be identified and treated. Make sure that you are tested for other imbalances such as hormonal imbalances, thyroid disorders, nutritional deficiencies, etc. These results also give you a good base-line for beginning your treatment programme. After three months, it is worthwhile rechecking these test results to see how you have improved.

Following the Anti-Candida Diet

The anti-Candida diet is an essential part of the treatment pro-gramme. There is no point trying to rebalance the internal environ-ment and killing the fungus, while at the same time feeding Candida its favourite foods.

It is important that you check if you have become allergic or sensi-tive to certain foods. This involves taking a food intolerance test, and then avoiding these foods for at least three months. During the three-month break from the foods to which you are sensitive, you should ensure that you rotate your diet every four days. For example, you may eat fish on Day 1, chicken on Day 2, lamb on Day 3 and beef on Day 4, then back to fish on Day 1 again. This should be done with all foods, including carbohydrates, fruits and vegetables. A nutritionist can design a good food-rotation plan for you.

An important point to mention, which many people do not recog-nize, is that Candida cannot effectively be treated through diet alone. German physicians have noted that by simply starving the Candida you effectively drive it deeper into the walls of the intestines. It has been suggested that this may occur because Candida can adapt to its deprivation of sugars by digesting the proteins in the cell walls of the intestine. You need to follow the entire treatment programme to combat Candida infection successfully.

The anti-Candida diet is discussed briefly in Chapter Five, but you are strongly advised to consult a qualified nutritionist for dietary advice, or at least buy a book Candida Diet Book.

On the face of it the anti-Candida diet may look very frugal and dull, but with the good advice of a nutritionist or a diet book you will discover that it can be both delicious and rewarding. Bear in mind the good news, your skin and hair will glow, you will probably lose excess fat without ever feeling hungry, and you will be eating your way back to health!

Taking Anti-fungal Medications

This is an area where you can choose to employ either orthodox medications or natural anti-fungal treatments. Both choices are effective, and below you will find an outline of some of the more popular choices.

If you choose to use orthodox medications you will need a prescription from your doctor. This might prove difficult if your doctor does not agree with your diagnosis of Candida. As mentioned earlier in this book, Candida is still a contentious subject in orthodox medical circles. If your doctor refuses to entertain the idea that you might have Candida, then you might get a better response by consulting a doctor who is trained in both orthodox and complementary medicine.

Conventional anti-fungal drugs are effective and easy to administer. The disadvantage of orthodox medicines is that they are unlikely to be able to provide you with the other 'tools' required to treat the environment of the body, these medicines only kill the fungus they don't rebalance the environment. Bear in mind also that some of these conventional drugs may produce unwanted side effects.

Whether you choose to use orthodox or complementary medicines is a decision that only you can make. Some of the side effects of anti-fungal medications include nausea, vomiting, diarrhea, abnormal liver functions, skin rashes, toxicity of the kidneys, headaches, amongst others. Details of specific side effects to particular medications can be obtained from books such as The British National Formulary.

The next two pages show tables outlining the most commonly used anti-fungal medications currently used in the treatment of Candidiasis by the orthodox medical profession.

Name of Drug	Uses	Side-effects
Clotrimazole (also known as Canesten) **Econazole** (also known as Ecostatin, Gyno-Pevaryl) **Fenticonazole** (also known as Lomexin) **Miconazole** (also known as Gyno-Daktarin) **Nystatin** (also known as Nystan)	<u>For vulval and vaginal Candida</u> Used as creams and pessaries Treatment may need to be extended for 6 months.	Occasional local irritation
Clotrimazole (Canesten) **Econazole** (Ecostatin, Pevaryl) **Ketoconazole** (Nizoral) **Miconazole** (Daktarin) **Sulconazole** (also known as Exelderm) **Nystatin** (also known as Nystaform)	<u>Anti-fungal preparations for the skin</u> Used as creams and powders	Occasional mild burning, redness and itching of the skin.
Amphotericin (also known as Fungilin)	<u>For candida of the mouth and thoat</u> Not absorbed from the gut, so taken as lozenges or a liquid	Mild disturbances in the gut
Nystatin (Nystan)	As above	Irritation of the mouth
Miconazole (Daktarin)	Taken as a gel	Nausea vomiting, diarrhoea, rarely allergic reactions
Fluconazole	See Below	See below

Name of Drug	Uses	Side-effects
	For systemic and intestinal Candida	
Amphotericin (also known as Fungilin, Fungizone, Abelcet, AmBisome, Amphocil)	For severe Candida. Given by mouth or injection	Side-effects are common and severe, including nausea, vomiting, diarrhoea, gut pain, fever, headaches, muscle and joint pain, disturbances in kidney function, disturbances of the heart, blood disorders, loss of hearing, double vision, spasms, abnormal liver function.
Flucytosine (also known as Ancotil)	For severe Candida. Given by injection	Nausea, vomiting, diarrhoea, rashes, confusion, hallucinations, spasms, headaches, drowsiness, vertigo, changes in liver function, blood disorders.
Fluconazole (also known as Diflucan)	Given by mouth or injection for systemic Candida	Nausea, gut discomfort, diarrhoea, flatulence, headache, rash, vomiting, dizziness, loss of hair, itchiness, high cholesterol.

Reproduced with kind permission from the British National Formulary, 44, Sept 2002.

Natural Anti-fungal Medications

An alternative to mainstream anti-fungal medication is to use natural anti-fungal treatments. These are very effective – in some cases even more so than synthetic drugs, because their natural chemical make-up is so complex that it is difficult for the fungus to develop resistance to them. Natural medicines also have the advantage of not being as toxic to the body as orthodox medications can be.

Garlic (Allium sativum)

As well as being one of the strongest anti-fungal agents available, garlic also reduces blood sugar levels, thus making it one of the most useful anti-Candida agents available.

It is quite possible to eat just raw cloves of garlic, but many people find this completely unpalatable. Garlic is best taken three times a day, with each meal, because it can make you feel quite nauseous when eaten on an empty stomach. You can choose to chop it and swallow with water, or include it in your meal as a salad dressing, crushed over baked potatoes or a hot steak, in tzatziki, or stirred into soup. Mediterranean people eat raw garlic rubbed onto rough toast or bread, topped with olive oil and tomatoes. However you choose to eat your garlic, it must be eaten in its raw state, as cooking destroys the active ingredient.

Alternatively, you can take garlic capsules, but not the deodorized or odourless garlic. Unfortunately it is the smelly component of the garlic which has the anti-fungal actions.

Side-effects: Ingestion of garlic will lead to a strong odour on the breath or body, however, if you take garlic before bed, you breathe off most of the odours during the night. Occasionally, garlic can cause irritation of the gut wall, flatulence, and inflammation of the nasal passages, asthma or eczema. Of greater concern is the fact that garlic thins the blood, and very large quantities may result in prolonged bleeding. The herb should not be taken by people taking anti-coagulant medication such as warfarin or aspirin.

Aloe vera Barbadensis or Capensis

Aloe vera juice is another plant extract with multiple actions to treat Candida. The most common use for aloe in China is as an anti-fungal agent, while in the West we focus mainly on its healing properties. Taken internally, aloe can be used to help eradicate Candida fungus and heal the gastric mucosa in the gut wall.

Aloe vera juice is best taken on an empty stomach so that it has the best opportunity to come into contact with the gastric wall. There are two types of Aloe juice. The whole-leaf extract is used for people suffering from constipation, as it has a laxative effect. The filleted aloe vera juice does not have this laxative effect, and is used entirely for its healing properties.

Side-effects: Very rarely, people may experience a stinging sensation when applying the gel onto their skin. People who drink the whole leaf juice extract are likely to experience cramping and diarrhoea, so rather focus on the filleted leaf extract, or a product which is 'Anthraquinone-free'. Pregnant and breast feeding women should avoid drinking the juice, but may use the gel topically.

Pau D'Arco/Lapacho (Tabebuia impeteginosa)

This herbal medicine comes from the inner bark of a South American tree. The bark is tremendously anti-fungal, and also has the effect of toning the immune system. In my experience it is best taken as a tea in combination with other herbs, where it can wash through the intestines and come into contact with the fungus as well as being absorbed into the bloodstream.

Myrrh (Commiphora molmol)

Myrrh is the brittle gum resin taken from the fissures in the bark of the myrrh bush. It has been used for thousands of years in the holy waters of the Jews, and was used for embalming by the ancient Egyptians. Myrrh is a potent anti-fungal agent and also has the effect of improving digestion by increasing the flow of digestive juices. Because in its natural state myrrh is a brittle lump of resin, it is best taken as a tincture (alcohol extract), but should be used in very small quantities.

Side-effects: No adverse effects are known when taken in therapeutic doses, however, this herb should not be taken during pregnancy.

Oregano (Origanum vulgare)

Oregano is a herb containing a volatile oil with powerful anti-fungal properties. It is possible to take oregano as a tea or tincture. This would be effective, but the most powerful form would be as an essential oil capsule. Biocare supply essential oil of oregano in a pre-prepared capsule complex (Oregano Complex), which also contains other anti-fungal agents such as oil of cloves, ginger and artemesia.

Side-effects: Although there are no known side-effects, this essential oil, as well as the Oregano complex should not be used during pregnancy or whilst breast feeding. You should never take essential oils internally, unless they have been specifically formulated by a qualified professional.

Caprylic Acid
Caprylic acid is a fatty acid derived from coconuts. Caprylic acid has been shown to be an effective anti-fungal agent, while at the same time not adversely affecting the friendly gut bacteria. Caprylic acid can be bought from Biocare in three strengths as Mycropryl 250mg (for children), Mycropryl 400mg and Mycropryl 680mg.

Grapefruit Seed Extract (Citracidal)
Grapefruit seed extract is an immensely powerful anti-fungal agent, and is commonly used for the treatment of Candida. I do not choose to prescribe this agent because, in the past, my patients have described it as 'too rough on the gut'. It is an extraordinarily abrasive agent, and there was an alarming case when someone even bled from the bowel for 10 days after taking the lowest recommended dose. Grapefruit seed extract has another disadvantage of killing off the friendly bacteria in the gut, so it really seems to be too harsh an agent to be of much use internally.

Externally, however, grapefruit seed extract does have some very good uses. It can be applied to stubborn fungal nail infections, and can be used to wash the socks of those who suffer from nail infections so that the spores are not transmitted back to the feet. Grapefruit seed extract can also be used as an anti-fungal agent when washing the fridge and around the sink – even vegetables and fruits can be dipped in a diluted solution to help eradicate fungal spores.

Oregon Grape (Berberis aquifolium)
Berberis is the inner bark of a spiny bush which contains a constituent called berberine, shown to be active against Candida as well as other disease-forming bacteria. It also contains hydrastine, an alkaloid which has the action of healing the mucous membranes of the body.

Berberis also acts on the liver to aid the detoxification process, and aids digestion by encouraging the secretion of gastric juices. Berberis can be taken either in the form of a tea, a tincture, or as a complex from Biocare, which also contains Pau D'Arco and garlic.

Side-effects: Overdose may result in nosebleeds, stupor, vomiting, diarrhoea and kidney irritation. This herb should not be taken during pregnancy.

Cinnamon (Cinnamomum zeylanicum)

This delicious kitchen spice has a wide range of applications in the treatment of Candida. It is an anti-fungal agent, but is also used by medical herbalists to treat nausea and diarrhoea. Cinnamon has an astringent effect on the tissues it comes into contact with, and therefore, taken as a tea or tincture, can contribute towards healing the leaky gut caused by Candida overgrowth. It also helps to treat the nausea associated with Candida, as well as helping to kill the fungus. Cinnamon has a naturally sweet taste, and this, combined with vanilla essence and FOS (see page 89), is an indispensable combination of ingredients when you feel the urge for something sweet!

The easiest way to ingest cinnamon is to pop a quill of the bark into a cup of boiling water with a few slices of fresh ginger and a slice of lemon, and sip as a delicious herbal tea. Alternatively, you can sprinkle powdered cinnamon over porridge or rice.

Side-effects: Taken as a kitchen herb, there are no side-effects, or known adverse reactions.

Olive Oil (Olea europa)

Olive oil contains a substance known as oleic acid. This constituent has the ability to interfere with the transformation of Candida from its innocuous yeast form into the invasive fungal form. Olive oil should be taken into the diet in its raw state, and you should have about six teaspoonfuls a day. As olive oil is used as a laxative in the Mediterranean, if you wish to avoid this effect, divide the doses into two teaspoonfuls three times a day. Olive oil can be included in your diet as a salad dressing, poured over soup, or simply by dipping bread into it and eating this with a little raw garlic.

Side-effects: Generally, this oil is completely safe to take internally, however, there have been cases when gallstone sufferers have suffered from gall-bladder colic as a result of taking olive oil.

Biotin

Biotin is one of the B vitamins. It is important in that, like olive oil, it helps to prevent the Candida converting from the yeast form into the fungal form.

Cautions: There are no known toxic effects from taking biotin. Be aware that raw-egg white deactivates the body's biotin.

Essential Oils

Essential oils are very powerful anti-fungal agents as they are the concentrated version of the herbal extracts. Essential oils are too potent to take internally, unless formulated by a trained professional. However, it is possible to include a little aromatherapy for the external treatment of thrush or fungal skin and nail infections. You can mix 2ml of the oils listed below with 100ml of a base oil, and this mixture can then be used in the bath or as a massage.

A soothing recipe for thrush is to add 20 drops of tea tree oil to a 60ml pot of aloe vera gel. Five drops of German chamomile essential oil will add a lovely anti-inflammatory effect. Stir vigorously, until well mixed. This can be applied directly to the vulva, vagina or penis to help to combat thrush. Keep this in the fridge for an extra soothing effect. Do not use this recipe if pregnant or breast feeding.

Anti-fungal essential oils include:

Plant Name	Safety Data
Tea tree (*Melaleuca alternifolia*)	Non-toxic and non-irritant. Possible sensitization in some individuals
Oregano (*Origanum vulgare*)	No health hazards or side-effects known
Thyme (*Thymus vulgaris*)	May contain large amounts of toxic components. Use only in small quantities
Lemongrass (*Cymbopogon citras*)	Non-toxic and non-irritant. Possible sensitization in some individuals
Palmarosa (*Cymbopogon martinii*)	Non-toxic, non-irritant, non-sensitizing
Myrrh (*Commiphora molmol*)	Do not use during pregnancy. Use only in small doses
Lemon-scented Eucalyptus (*Eucalyptus citriodora*)	Non-toxic and non-irritant. Possible sensitization in some individuals

Just bear in mind that Candida is the master of adaptation. To help to prevent the Candida from developing resistance to your anti-fungal regime, alternate your anti-fungal medications every two weeks.

Anti-fungal Foods
Olive oil
Garlic, leeks, onions
Herbs and spices such as thyme, oregano, turmeric and cinnamon.
Teas such as cinnamon, Pau D'Arco

An Anti-fungal Snack
1 cup of cooked brown rice
1 clove of crushed garlic
2 tablespoons of extra virgin olive oil
¼ of a lemon, squeezed into juice
Add variety by throwing in chopped tomatoes, tuna or nuts. Mix all the ingredients together and enjoy at least once a day!

Healing a Leaky Gut Wall

Healing a leaky gut wall is an extremely important part of the anti-Candida treatment programme. A leaky gut allows undigested food particles to enter the bloodstream, causing food sensitivities and allergies to develop, and putting strain on the immune system. It also allows micro-organisms to enter, placing the immune system under even greater strain.

The following supplements can be used to help heal the intestinal wall.

Butyric Acid
Butyric acid is one of the primary sources of energy for the rapidly dividing cells lining the wall of the intestinal tract, and thus is extremely useful in helping to improve the integrity of the gut wall. Biocare supplies a Butyric acid complex which has been formulated to ensure availability over a long period of time.

L Glutamine
Glutamine is an amino acid which also provides fuel for the rapidly

dividing tissues of the intestinal tract. Normally there is sufficient glutamine in the body to meet the demands required for the fuelling of new intestinal cells, but when the body has an increased turnover of intestinal cells, as in leaky gut syndrome, then supplementation of this amino acid is advisable. Lamberts supplies L Glutamine in capsule form, and suggests taking 1000mg per day half an hour before meals. This product should not be used by women who are pregnant or breast feeding.

N-Acetyl Glucosamine

N-Acetyl Glucosamine (NAG) is another supplement required for the formation of the matrix, which binds the cells of the gut wall.

Fructo-oligosaccharides (FOS)

Sweet-tasting FOS is one of the mainstays of the Candida treatment programme. FOS is known as a prebiotic which is a substance needed to feed the friendly bacteria (probiotics) in order for them to proliferate. It is derived from fruit sugar, but instead of being bad for you, in this case it is good for your anti-Candida programme. FOS resists being broken down in the gut as well as being transported across the gut barrier into the bloodstream. Therefore, FOS is able to supply food to the friendly bacteria and encourage their proliferation, without affecting blood sugar levels or encouraging the growth of yeast. When FOS is fermented by the bacteria it produces butyric acid, and thereby also contributes to the healing of the gut membrane. FOS is available through Biocare or Lamberts. Beware of eating too much FOS, because it can cause gas. If you find this happening, cut back your dose.

Aloe Vera Juice

As mentioned above, aloe juice is one of the best healers of the gut wall, and is safe enough to be taken three times a day for an unlimited period. Take 10ml three times a day on an empty stomach.

Marigold (Calendula officinalis)

The beautiful orange petals of Calendula flowers are one of the great healers of the intestinal wall, and absolutely invaluable when treating a leaky gut. Calendula is also an anti-fungal agent, as well as acting on the liver to aid the detoxification process.

Side-effects: None reported

Glycyrrhiza Glabra (Liquorice)

Liquorice root has a significant anti-inflammatory effect on the gastric membrane, as well as contributing towards the healing of any lesions in this area. It is 50 times sweeter than sugar as very little is needed. As well as its healing effects liquorice provides some welcome sweetness to herbal teas. Liquorice is very well known to herbalists for its positive restoring effect on the adrenal glands. In Candida, this is certainly an action which is called for.

Side-effects: Excessive or prolonged use of liquorice has resulted in some individuals developing a condition known as 'hyperaldosteronism'. This condition results in increased sodium and water retention, increased blood pressure, amongst other problems, however this condition will resolve within a month of ceasing to take the herb. Liquorice should be completely avoided by individuals who suffer from cardiac conditions, high blood pressure, and also be those who have a blood sugar imbalance. It should also be avoided by pregnant and breast feeding women.

Chamomile (Matracaria recutita)

German chamomile is known as the 'Mother of the Gut'. The flowers contain volatile oils known as bisabolol and azulenes which have a wide range of medicinal actions when released by hot water as in a tea. These oils have the effect of reducing the painful inflammation of leaky gut syndrome, and healing the mucous membrane of the intestinal tract. In addition they relieve spasm, calm the mind and have a mild anti-fungal action.

Ask a herbalist to combine a tea-mixture of German chamomile flowers, calendula petals and liquorice chips. Use this mixture to make a soothing herbal tea specifically to heal the leaky gut. Add 1 tablespoon of the tea per cup of boiling water, steep for 5 minutes, strain and pour. Drink this tea three times a day.

Side-effects: Chamomile should be avoided by those people allergic to flowers of the daisy family (Asteracea), as it may provoke an allergic attack.

Foods that Help Heal a Leaky Gut

Anthrocyanidins are components of a plant pigment group known as flavonoids, and are used therapeutically by medical herbalists and nutritionists for their ability to heal fragility and leakiness in tissues. Plants rich in these pigments include black grapes (with the skin on), blueberries and cranberries. These fruits can be combined with some rice milk, FOS and milled oats to form a deliciously healing smoothie.

Repopulating the Intestine with Probiotics

Candida is a form of gross dysbiosis. Dysbiosis refers to a condition when the flora of the intestine are out of balance. This can happen with any of the flora of the gut, but in this case it is that the Candida yeast that is dominating the friendly bacteria. The balance needs to be corrected if you are to gain health again.

Probiotics come in capsules or powders made up of live human strain friendly bacteria, which are supplied to the intestines with the intention of repopulating the gut with friendly bacteria. By introducing billions of viable friendly bacteria, you immediately change the ratio of Candida to bacteria. The beneficial bacteria should also be encouraged by including in your repopulation regime prebiotics such as FOS, but most good probiotic formulas have FOS included in the capsule or powder. Once the flora balance is corrected, the bacteria can set about dominating the Candida and putting it back in its place, as well as synthesizing vital nutrients and vitamins.

A Word about Probiotics

There is a great inconsistency in the quality of probiotics available on the market. A study in 1996 showed that many 'acidophilus' products on the market did not match their claims of bacterial specifications, and were either inactive or contained fewer than 10 per cent of the declared dose of bacteria.

Criteria for a Good Commercial Preparation of Probiotics

- The bacteria should be human strain bacteria and not bovine strain bacteria
- The bacteria should be capable of attaching to the intestine wall
- The bacteria should be acid stable and capable of resisting stomach acids
- Both Lactobacillus acidophilus and Bifidobacteria should be

included in the product
- It is preferable if prebiotics such as FOS are included with the bacteria.
- Probiotic supplements should contain at least one billion viable friendly bacteria per daily dose.
- The product should have a shelf life which guarantees the bacteria are provided to the buyer in a live and viable state.
- The product should list an expiry date. Ref:BIOMED Newsletter Issue No. 10 Dec '94,Vol. 1, Number 1, Nov '89)
- The bacteria should be human-specific and capable of attaching to the gut lining.

A Recolonization Programme

Weeks 1– 2   Take a probiotic formulation which has between 20 billion and 30 billion viable bacteria per day. 'Replete' by Biocare provides 30 billion friendly bacteria in seven daily sachets.

Weeks 3 – 12   Take 4 billion bacteria per day, in two divided doses with meals, with breakfast and supper. Biocare's 'Bio-Acidophilus' provides the probiotics with the FOS in capsule form. Lambert's 'Acidophilus Extra' provides 4 billion viable bacteria, suitable for those intolerant to dairy products.

If FOS is not included in the formulation, then take a heaped teaspoon of the powder with each probiotic dose. Should you not be able to get hold of FOS, then psyllium seeds, pectin or aloe vera juice are good substitutes.

Aiding the Digestive Process

To benefit from the foods we eat, it is necessary that they are broken down fully into their component parts, so that the nutrients may be absorbed from the gut and utilized by the body to nourish and heal. The whole digestive system is disrupted by Candida, and this needs to be addressed as urgently as the Candida itself.

Poor enzymatic secretion has the following effects on the Candida sufferer:

- The food is not fully broken down into its component parts, and thus nutrients are unable to be utilized by the body, resulting in a state of malnutrition.
- Undigested food particles form a food substrate for the yeast to ferment, causing gas and bloating.
- Undigested food particles enter the bloodstream through the leaky gut and further deplete the immune system reserves by setting up allergic responses.
- A lack of digestive enzymes leads to indigestion and a feeling of excessive fullness and heaviness after a meal.

When a person is chronically ill, even their digestion packs up, so you need to help your body assimilate the nutrition from your food by providing digestive enzymes until such time as your body can start to produce its own again.

For the first month of the programme, take a plant-derived broad-spectrum digestive enzyme capsule at the start of each meal. These little capsules can be found at health food stores and should be taken with every meal to ensure that you receive your proper nourishment from your food. Also, if the food is broken down properly into its component parts, there is less of a chance of undigested food particles setting up further food sensitivities.

From the second month of the programme you can start to encourage your natural enzymatic secretion by placing a few drops of *Berberis aquifolium* (Oregon grape) on your tongue a few minutes before each meal. Berberis is a bitter herb that stimulates the digestive organs to secrete their own digestive juices.

Make sure that you chew your food thoroughly, as the food needs to be well mixed with the enzymes in order to be broken down sufficiently.

Pineapple and pawpaw both contain natural protein-digesting enzymes. Eating a few slices of one or the other at the start of a meal will help to encourage the digestion of proteins.

Herbs and spices such as ginger, garlic, turmeric, thyme and rosemary also encourage the secretion of digestive enzymes, so try to include these in your meals where possible.

Food-combining diets such as the Hay Diet aim to separate foods which require different digestive enzymes for their breakdown. When an acid and an alkali combine, you get a neutral environment, which does not digest any food at all. As a result you are left with undigested food putrefying in your intestinal tract, allowing toxins to leach back into your bloodstream, and also denying your body the nutrients it needs to survive and thrive. The Hay Diet suggests that you eat protein foods with vegetables and salads, and carbohydrate foods with vegetables and salads, but never protein and carbohydrates together.

Rest and Digest

There is much to be said for the old adage about not engaging in heated debates while eating. Eating in a stressful environment is not conducive to digestion, as the body is too busy preparing to fight or defend itself, so that the digestive system is put on hold until the stress has passed. When you eat your food in a restful state, the body is able to concentrate on the digestive process, and you enjoy your meal far more anyway.

Make sure that you are tested for nutritional deficiencies, and address these deficiencies with good quality nutritional supplements. Nutritional tests are available through a nutritionist, who can also provide you with the correct supplement programme.

Supporting Liver Function

The liver has so many jobs to do for the body. One of its major functions is to detoxify the blood. Candida presents a whole load of toxins to the body, and the liver has to deal with these on top of its normal toxic load. Among other functions, the liver is also involved in digestion, in maintaining normal blood sugar levels, and in the excretion of hormones. Traditional Chinese Medicine also states that the liver circulates the *Qi* (vital energy of the body). If *Qi* becomes sluggish or congested, then it stagnates, leading to a loss of energy. So it is clear from many perspectives that it is important to give your liver as much support as possible.

One of the best tonics for the liver is the seed of milk thistle (*Silybum marianum*). Milk thistle can be taken once a day in a capsule form, or as a tincture.

Another excellent liver-supporting herb is dandelion root (*Taraxacum officinalis radix*), which can be drunk as a substitute for coffee, or taken as a capsule or tincture.

The body eliminates toxins via the bowel, urine, skin and lungs, so other methods of detoxifying are also appropriate. A hot bath with 1kg of Epsom salts will allow you to sweat toxins out through the pores of your skin. Make sure you have a cool rinse or shower afterwards to wash the toxins off your skin. A sauna is another method of encouraging toxin elimination via the skin.

An aromatherapy massage with celery seed, carrot seed and juniper essential oils will encourage the flushing of the kidneys, and the elimination of toxins via the urine. Alternatively, you can drink a herbal tea of celery seeds, dandelion leaf and nettle to encourage elimination via the kidneys.

Colonic irrigation is a form of hydrotherapy which provides an excellent and instant method of detoxifying the bowel. Water is introduced into the bowel to flush out old sticky faecal matter and Candida, leaving the colon cleansed of toxins. At the end of the treatment, friendly bacteria are reintroduced into the empty bowel so that the ideal environment is maintained. See Useful Addresses at the back of the book for further details.

Foods to Support the Liver
Artichoke eaten steamed or grilled
Ginger as a tea with lemon and mint, or as a spice in stir-fries
Turmeric as a spice in curries
Oranges, lemons, mandarins – eaten fresh
Olive oil and olives
Dandelion root drunk as a coffee substitute
Milk thistle as a tea, tincture or in capsule form
Beetroot and carrot juice drink two glasses a day of home-made juice

Rebalancing Your Hormones

Before even starting to take hormonal herbs, it is vital that you get your female hormone levels tested so that you know which herbs are most appropriate. As you saw earlier in the book, some authorities suggest that progesterone may be the dominant factor, while others have noted that oestrogen is to blame. It is becoming clearer that as Candida is such a complex problem no single hormone can be blamed, and the likelihood is that it is a hormonal imbalance that needs to be addressed.

There are many herbs which have an effect on the hormones, but with each herb there are subtle differences. It is not advisable to use hormone-influencing herbs unless you really know what you are doing, because you could quite easily make your situation even worse. The skill and experience of a trained medical herbalist will safely determine which is the right herb for your particular case.

Herbs that Influence Progesterone
Vitex agnus castus
Please note that so-called 'Wild Yam natural progesterone cream' is not really very natural. In its natural state, Wild Yam (*Dioscorea villosa*) is actually an oestrogenic herb, but in the laboratory this steroid can be altered to mimic progesterone, and thus it exhibits a progesterogenic effect.

Herbs with an Oestrogenic Effect
Black cohosh (*Cimicifuga racemosa*)
Red clover (*Trifolium pratense*)
Herbs with a Positive Effect on the Adrenal Glands
Liquorice (*Glycyrrhiza glabra*)
Borage (*Borago officinalis*)

Treating Your Immune System

One of the reasons Candida is able to take hold is that the immune system may already be weakened. However, as you have seen, Candida also directly attacks the immune system by destroying the MALT immune tissues found on the lining of the gut wall. Candida also directly attacks the cellular arm of the immune system through toxin release, and causes further depletion of the humoral arm of the immune system through the antigen antibody complexes which have to be formed in response to the leaked undigested food particles.

Through healing the leaky gut and avoiding the foods to which you are sensitive, you have already gone a long way towards giving your immune system the break it needs so recovery can begin. But more can be done, and this is where herbs and nutritional supplements can really give your immune system the extra support necessary for recovery.

Some of these natural medications directly attack Candida, while others stimulate the immune system – but none of them should be used all the time. These remedies are far better if used for about six weeks before changing to another immune tonic. In this way the immune system has more global support, and also the fungus is unable to become resistant to any one remedy.

Echinacea (Echinacea purpurea/angustifolia)
This herb is well known for its immune-stimulating effects. There is controversy about how exactly this herb influences the immune system, but at least one respected reference suggests that the activity of Echinacea is directed towards cellular immunity. Some authorities strongly caution that Echinacea should not be used in auto-immune conditions or allergic subjects however, other research suggests that Echinacea is an immune tonic and that it would be indicated for these disorders. Many herbalists have found that patients with allergic conditions such as asthma and hay fever respond favourably to Echinacea, but this is a matter of personal experience by the medical herbalist.

It is well known that Echinacea should not be used for longer than six weeks before giving it a break and changing to another immune-toning herb.

Side-effects: As Echinacea is of the Asteraceae family, it would be prudent for those people who are allergic to other members of this daisy family of plants to avoid Echinacea. Echinacea should not be taken continuously for more than 6 weeks. Some scientists have theorised that Echinacea should be avoided in autoimmune diseases such as lupus and rheumatoid arthritis, however, this point is still being debated. Without sufficient evidence to suggest otherwise, it would be wise for pregnant and breast-feeding women to avoid taking this herb.

Huang Qi (Astragalus membranaceus)
Astragalus acts as a tonic to both the humoral and cellular arms of the immune system. One clinical study showed that a formula containing this herb improved the vigour, strength, sleep, appetite and vision in 507 subjects. In another study it raised and maintained white blood cell counts of patients with low cell counts. Chinese medical herbalists suggest that Huang Qi may be used by slicing the root and

cooking it with rice, to drink as a tea. Western medical herbalists will supply it as a tincture or in capsules.

Side-effects: No known side-effects

Chinese or Korean Ginseng (Panax ginseng)
Another well-known and deservedly respected herb, ginseng has many actions, among the most documented of which is its ability to improve the mental and physical stamina of both humans and animals. Ginseng has the effect of reducing the symptoms of depression and anxiety while at the same time toning the adrenal glands, which allows the person to adapt and recover effectively from stress. This amazing herb has been shown in numerous studies to provide considerable improvement to mood, mental performance and memory. It has also been shown repeatedly in studies to improve physical stamina, muscle strength and recovery time.

Ginseng protects the liver and is also protective against the effects of toxicity. It has also been shown to reduce blood sugar levels as well as enhance blood clearance of alcohol in humans. This is particularly relevant in Candida, as the yeast ferments sugars into alcohol, which might account for many of the symptoms of Candida. In terms of immunity, Ginseng enhances both humoral and cellular activity, and so all round this is a fabulous herb to use in the treatment of Candida.

Side-effects: Ginseng Abuse Syndrome exhibits symptoms, and thus the side effects of ginseng, to include increased blood pressure, diarrhoea, sleeplessness, nervousness, skin eruptions. Less commonly, other symptoms might include disturbances in menstruation, breast pain, depression and euphoria. Allergic reactions may include palpitations, sleeplessness, itchiness, headache, amongst others.
Ginseng should be avoided by those people taking MAOI's for depression, those with heart problems, high blood pressure, people taking steroidal drugs of any kind, and persons of nervous, tense or manic tendencies.

Siberian Ginseng (Eleuthrococcus senticosus)
This has similar effects to Panax ginseng, but is gentler. Medication with Eleuthrococcus also results in considerable improvement in mental and physical stamina, as well as the ability to cope with stress far more effectively. This ginseng also demonstrates immune-moderating effects, and particularly improves cellular immunity.

Siberian ginseng seems to have an interesting effect on the sex hormones in that it is able to bind with the receptors for progesterone and oestrogen; this may serve to help rebalance the hormonal system.

Please note that ginseng should not be used by people suffering from high blood pressure or poor sleep.

Side-effects: In studies, a very small percentage of people reported side effects, such as sleeplessness, shifts in heart rhythms, headaches, and increased blood pressure, however, these people were receiving very high doses of Siberian Ginseng.

Ashwaghanda/Indian Ginseng (Withania somnifera)

Withania is an important tonic, because unlike the Korean or Siberian ginsengs, which are stimulating in their actions, Withania improves stamina while at the same time relaxing the mind. It is particularly indicated for people suffering from debility and nervous exhaustion, and those suffering from long-term illness where inflammation is involved. Over time it has an immune-toning effect.

Garlic (Allium sativum)

Garlic must be one of the most useful herbs in the world. In the case of Candida, it has three major actions:

1. It is a direct anti-fungal, and thereby helps to kill off the fungus.
2. It contributes to improving cellular immunity.
3. It has blood sugar-lowering effects, and so helps to starve out the fungus, which relies on sugar for growth.

Side-effects: Ingestion of garlic will lead to a strong odour on the breath or body, however, if you take garlic before bed, you breathe off most of the odours during the night. Occasionally, garlic can cause irritation of the gut wall, flatulence, and inflammation of the nasal passages, asthma or eczema. Of greater concern is the fact that garlic thins the blood, and very large quantities may result in prolonged bleeding. The herb should not be taken by people taking anti-coagulant medication such as warfarin or aspirin.

Nutritional Supplements that Improve Immune Function

Buffered Vitamin C is an antioxidant which helps to protect the body against toxins, cancer and infection, and helps to enhance immunity. Vitamin C may irritate the stomach and cause symptoms of diarrhoea. To help prevent this, use esterified vitamin C, which is gentler on the stomach and better absorbed. Dose: 1 gram per day.

Side-effects: No known side effects at the therapeutic dose

Selenium is an antioxidant and enhances the immune system by protecting against the formation of free radicals. Dose: 200mcg/day.

Zinc fights free radicals and promotes a healthy immune system. It is best absorbed in citrate form at a dose of 50mg/day.

Side-effects: No known side effects when taken in therapeutic doses.

Summary

Weeks 1 –2

1. Get tested.

2. Start the anti-Candida diet.

3. Repopulate with probiotics:
   - Take 20 billion bacteria per day with meals.
   - Take 15 grams of FOS per day in divided doses three times a day, if it is not included in your probiotic capsules.

4. Help the digestive process:
   - Take broad-spectrum digestive enzymes with every meal.
   - Place about 10 drops of Oregon grape tincture on your tongue 10 minutes before each meal.

Weeks 3 –12

1. Continue with the anti-Candida diet.

2. Take anti-fungal medications. Remember to alternate these anti-fungal remedies fortnightly:
   - Garlic – 3 cloves of undeodorized capsules per day with each meal
   - Oregano complex as directed on the bottle
   - Myrrh 20 drops in water three times a day before meals
   - Pau D'Arco 3 to 5 cups of tea per day

- Oregon grape 20 drops three times a day
- Cinnamon in tea or tincture three times a day
- Biotin – 300mcg per day

3. Heal the leaky gut, using the following herbs and supplements interchangeably:
   - Butyric acid as directed on the bottle
   - L Glutamine as directed on the bottle
   - N-Acetyl Glucosamine (NAG) as directed on the bottle
   - Aloe vera juice 10ml three times a day before meals
   - Marigold, chamomile and liquorice tea – three to five times a day

4. Repopulate with probiotics:
   - Take 4 billion bacteria per day.
   - Take 15 grams of FOS per day, if it is not included in your probiotic capsules.

5. Help the digestive process:
   - Take broad-spectrum digestive enzymes with every meal for weeks 3 and 4, and for longer if you require it.
   - Place about 10 drops of Oregon grape on your tongue 10 minutes before each meal.
   - Eat a few slices of raw pineapple or pawpaw before each meal to help encourage protein digestion if your diet allows fruit
   - Get tested for nutritional deficiencies and take the relevant supplements to redress the balance.

6. Support liver function:
   - Milk thistle dose as directed on the bottle, twice a day
   - Dandelion root tea twice a day

   Other detoxification methods:
   - Epsom salt baths
   - Aromatherapy massage with celery seed, carrot seed, and juniper essential oils
   - Colonic irrigation
   - Saunas and steam baths

7. Rebalance your hormones:
   - The herb with a progesterone-balancing effect is *Vitex agnus castus*

The herbs with oestrogenic balancing effects include:
- Black cohosh take as directed on bottle or by your herbalist
- Liquorice take as directed on bottle or by your herbalist
- Red clover take as directed on bottle or by your herbalist

8. Treat the immune system by alternating between using the following herbs:
- Echinacea
- Astragulus
- Korean ginseng
- Siberian ginseng
- Ashwaghanda

Use the following nutritional supplements:
- Vitamin C 1 g per day
- Zinc citrate 50mg day

Week 12 Onwards

Depending on how severely you have been affected by Candida, you may or may not have started to notice that you are feeling better by now.

Retake your diagnostic tests to see how much you have improved, and decide whether you need to continue with all parts of the programme. Adjust the programme accordingly.

- Once your symptoms have eased off, you can start slowly to re-introduce foods to which you were sensitive. If you react to certain foods, avoid them again. You are advised to remain off the foods to which you are sensitive for at least three months. Do make sure that you have an adequate diet to avoid malnutrition.
- It is possible that your leaky gut is now healed, but it is worth your while to continue using chamomile and calendula tea for a few more months.
- If your menstrual symptoms are better controlled, you can wean yourself off the hormone-balancing herbs. If you are showing improvement but are not fully well, then continue to treat yourself. If you have seen no improvement, then see a herbalist for this problem.

- You are probably OK to stop taking specific liver-enhancing medicines now.
- You can try to use fewer anti-fungal and probiotic medications, and see if your symptoms flare up again. If they do, continue with these remedies. If you are OK, just continue to tone your immune system.
- Take care that you do not indulge in Candida-encouraging foods.
- Avoid at all costs the original cause of your illness.

In the next chapter we'll take a closer look at Step 10 in the anti-Candida programme: redressing your lifestyle.

Chapter Eleven

Adopting a Candida-free Lifestyle

Keeping Your Home Mould-free

It is common with people who suffer from Candida to also be allergic to other environmental moulds or fungi. You will know if you are sensitive to moulds if your symptoms flare up during cold and damp weather, when you are near compost heaps, or when you are in cold and dank environments. If your symptoms arise under these conditions, then you need to do all that you can to avoid them and eradicate them from your environment. One of the best things you can do is to keep your home very well ventilated and cool, so make sure to throw open all the windows for at least an hour a day, and keep the central heating as low as you and your family can cope with. In your own bedroom, try not to have the heating on at all.

Moulds thrive in dark, damp and warm conditions, so that makes the kitchen and bathroom two prime areas for fungal growth.

In the Kitchen

Mould can easily grow in the kitchen, especially in places like the refrigerator, around the sink and plugholes, in fruit bowls and on wooden spoons and chopping boards. All surfaces should regularly be cleaned with an anti-mould agent. If you prefer to use a natural agent, this is where grapefruit seed extract really comes into its own.

The spores of fungi also float about in the air, so to avoid contamination of food, dip all fruit and vegetables in a solution of grapefruit seed extract and water before eating. Leftovers should immediately be covered with foil or plastic wrap and frozen to minimize contamination with spores.

All foods containing fungi, such as mushrooms, brewer's yeast, etc., should be thrown out of the home

In the Bathroom

All surfaces in the bathroom should be regularly washed down with an anti-fungal agent, and shower curtains should be washed once a week to eliminate fungal spores. Prime areas for mould growth are around the bath plugholes, taps, within the overflow outlet, and around the edges of window frames.

The bathroom is a hot moist room, so make sure that it is well ventilated during the day to avoid the build-up of unseen mouldy growth.

Other Areas of Your Home
Conservatories and greenhouses are warm and moist, and therefore have huge potential for fungal growth, so bear this in mind and keep them well ventilated to avoid the growth of moulds. The garden is another area for potential growth of moulds. Try to keep areas like the compost heap as far away from the house as is possible. Also try to make sure that autumn leaves are swept up quickly and not allowed to lie on the ground and become mouldy.

On Holiday

After all the work you will have put into treating your Candida, the last thing you want to do is mess it up on holiday. Many people relax their regime when away, and as a result their symptoms flare up and they don't enjoy their holiday. Try as best you can to avoid slipping off the anti-Candida diet. Find out as much as you can about the region to which you are travelling, and if chances are that you will have to live off lots of white bread and pastries, for instance, then prepare for this by taking plenty of rice crackers, etc. with you.

Phone the hotel and airline ahead of time, and find out about their menus. You could mention that you are on a special diet, and ask if they will cater for you. Most hotels will not have any idea about an anti-Candida diet, but if you ask for a menu for people with diabetes or a wheat-/dairy-free menu, you are likely to have a better response.

The ideal location for a holiday is the desert or a Mediterranean climate because of their dryness. The Mediterranean also has the advantage of including plenty of garlic and onions in its traditional cuisine, and a wide variety of delicious dishes which will not interfere with your anti-Candida diet. You might even pick up some good recipe tips.

Be aware that indoor swimming pool areas can also be good breeding grounds for moulds, so try to find a place where you can swim outdoors or in the sea.

If you feel nervous about being away from home, then take mini-weekend breaks, or indulge in day-breaks to spas or yoga centres, until your confidence builds up sufficiently to take a longer break from home.

Treat Yourself

Most people in the Western world tend to 'treat' themselves by indulging in refined foods. Some people choose chocolate while others indulge in alcohol. Whatever the case, the anti-Candida diet puts a very strict end to these treats, and this can leave you feeling really bereft and punished for being ill. For this reason it is very important to find other ways of rewarding yourself. You might like to book a facial or pedicure at a beauty salon, buy a lovely book, or take a class in painting or some form of exercise. Fill this gap in your life with something that you have always really wanted to do, but never got around to. After all, you never know where this may lead you!

It is equally important to give yourself time out to rest and recover. You can't get better unless you rest your body and your mind, which allows the recovery process to take place. This timeout might take the form of a Buddhist retreat, a spa weekend, an hour alone in your bedroom every evening, a regular yoga class, or a daily early-morning meditation. Whatever form of rest you choose make sure that you get it.

Your Clothing

You need to keep yourself as cool and dry as possible, so do be careful to wear only natural fibres such as cotton, linen, silk and wool. Skirts are cooler than trousers as they allow a better air-flow between your legs. Many women find that nylon tights are the worst things for thrush, and choose to wear stockings instead. Some women even prefer not to wear knickers at all, or to use the crotchless type. While it may take some getting used to, these precautions do allow your genital area to remain cooler, with less chance of thrush developing.

Another thing to be fastidious about is making sure that your clothes are bone dry before putting them back in your wardrobe or drawers. It is so easy not to notice that clothes are just slightly damp when they are put into those dark, warm wardrobes and drawers, which will allow mould to insidiously take hold. Using a very hot wash and tumble dryer will contribute towards destroying fungal spores, as will ironing. You can also sprinkle a few drops of anti-fungal essential oils in your drawers or on a card to hang in your wardrobe.

Your Friends and Family

One of the most uncomfortable aspects of developing a chronic illness such as Candida is dealing with how friends and family perceive you. When someone is ill, we expect to see a wound, or at least have a diagnosis, but with Candida you often don't even *look* ill, although you are. As conventional medicine rarely recognizes Candida outside the realms of AIDS or diabetes, etc., you can be left feeling like a fraud, and uninformed people might even accuse you of being a hypochondriac.

It is important that you don't let this type of attitude get you down. You need the support of people close to you, so speak to them about the illness, tell them how it feels to have Candida, and how it feels to be on the treatment programme demystify the illness for them.

Also, don't be afraid to ask for help. When you are feeling very ill, your mind is foggy or you are physically exhausted, you will need all the help you can get with housework, shopping, remembering the medication, etc. Some very kind partners or parents even support the Candida sufferer by also sticking to the anti-Candida diet. If you don't have someone to help you, then you may find that keeping a 'things to-do' diary helps you to plan your day and cope with forgetfulness.

Many people find that support groups are invaluable for maintaining morale. In these groups you can talk to people who also have Candida but may be some way down the line towards better health. They can offer encouragement at crucial times when you may feel like giving up. Support groups also are pretty good about feeding you the latest information regarding new research and treatment methods.

Your Sexual Relationships

Many women find that they develop thrush and vaginitis (inflammation of the vagina and vulva) immediately after sexual intercourse. This understandably makes these women very reluctant to make love with their partners, which can, unfortunately, undermine the relationship. A good relationship with your partner is very important for many reasons, but purely from a Candida perspective, a happy relationship is invaluable both of in terms your emotional well-being and to help you cope with the rigours of the treatment programme.

The reason why women develop thrush after intercourse is that the vagina is naturally an acid environment, and this is conducive to the health of the friendly bacteria which reside there and keep the Candida under control. When a man ejaculates into the vagina, his semen changes the pH of the vagina towards a more alkaline state. The semen remains in the vagina for some hours after the event, and the friendly bacteria suffer as a result, while the yeast flourishes. It seems that some women are more sensitive to this effect than others, but this certainly does not mean that you cannot enjoy a healthy sexual relationship.

It is important that immediately after sex you should have a cool bath or vaginal douche, to wash the semen out of your vagina. By adding a little vinegar to the water, or squeezing a lemon under the water between your legs, you are restoring the pH to a more acid environment again. Keep your bath cool, as hot baths can aggravate the condition.

You can also boost the friendly bacterial populations of your vagina by rolling a tampon in some plain live yoghurt and inserting it for a few minutes. Alternatively, you can break open an acidophilus capsule and mix it with a little aloe vera gel, dip a tampon in this mixture and insert into the vagina.

It is extremely important that your partner is treated for thrush at the same time as yourself. Men rarely exhibit symptoms of a yeast infection, although they frequently carry the yeast and reinfect their partner every time they make love. Men are generally not very happy about the idea that they might be contributing to your thrush, and might even take umbrage, believing that you are accusing them of giving you a sexually transmitted disease. Choose a good moment and gently explain why it is that you develop thrush after intercourse. He doesn't need to do very much. If you make him an anti-fungal gel to apply to his penis before intercourse, it will go a long way to helping prevent you developing thrush and preserving a happy sexual relationship.

Thrush Gel
Add 10 drops of tea tree essential oil and 10 drops of palmarosa essential oil to 60ml of aloe vera gel. Mix well and apply to the penis before intercourse. This gel can also be introduced to the vagina by adding it to your bath. Make sure to do a patch test on the inside of the wrist before applying this gel to delicate tissues.

You might also like to consider using a condom, which would immediately prevent the change of pH by acting as a barrier between the vagina and the semen.

If the Pill is to blame for starting your Candida problem, then of course you would be advised to try another form of contraception. Naturally this is a decision that should be made by both partners.

What about Oral Thrush?
Thrush in the mouth manifests as white plaques on the inside of the lips and cheeks. These plaques can be scraped off, but they can often bleed. Oral thrush is a sign of widespread Candida, but can be quite easily controlled as long as you bear in mind that you need to treat not just your mouth but your whole body.

One of the simplest things you can do is to start to use tea tree toothpaste. Tea tree, being an anti-fungal agent as well as an anti-bacterial agent, will protect your teeth from the harmful effects of bacteria as well as going some way towards dealing with the fungal plaques in your mouth. If you don't find that a tea tree toothpaste is enough to combat oral thrush, then you can make up a powerfully effective myrrh mouthwash.

Oral Thrush Mouthwash
20 drops of Myrrh (*Commiphora molmol*) tincture in a glass of water.

Rinse your mouth and gargle with this mouthwash for at least 3 minutes twice a day, spitting out after rinsing. Try not to eat or drink anything for 10 minutes after rinsing to allow the myrrh to do its work.

The Die-off Effect

The 'die-off effect' is a common side-effect of an anti-Candida treatment programme. When the yeast starts to die, its cell bodies release toxins, which literally poison your body so that you can feel even worse than you did before you started the treatment programme.

Another reason for this effect is that the anti-Candida diet is so pure that you will go through a natural detoxification process. The toxins which have been stored in your fatty tissues will be released into your bloodstream and this will also contribute to the uncomfortable effects. This is the time when many Candida sufferers give up the treatment programme because they just can't bear the idea of feeling worse before they get better.

The good news is that the die-off effect is proof that the yeast is dying and that the treatment is working. After this initial period, which may last between three days and two weeks, you will experience much better mental clarity and increased energy.

Die-off Symptoms
- headaches
- muscle and joint pain
- increased fatigue
- abnormal sweating, discharges from the skin and unusual body odour
- changes in bowel habit
- nausea
- mucus
- foggy head
- flu-like symptoms

The die-off effect is by no means inevitable. There are things that can be done to minimize the effects. Some therapists recommend that their patients start the anti-Candida diet two weeks before taking the other medications, so that the yeast can become starved and weakened. By doing this, some of the yeast will die through starvation and so the release of toxins will be more gradual, and the body will be better able to deal with the process. If the die-off effect continues while you are taking the anti-fungal medications, then cut back on these remedies until the symptoms ease then you can gradually build them up again to an effective dose.

The liver is the detox centre of the body, so it is important to give this organ all the support you can. Milk thistle is a fabulous liver-supporting herb, and is specifically used to help the liver deal with toxins.

Another herb that will help tremendously during the die-off period is ginger. Ginger increases bile flow, which flushes toxins from the liver. Ginger is also a wonderful anti-nausea herb. One of the best ways of taking ginger is in a tea.

Ginger Tea

5 slices of fresh ginger root (don't worry about peeling the root)

1 slice of lemon

1 cup of boiling water

You can also add an organic peppermint teabag or a sprig of mint to the tea.

Steep together for 5 minutes and sip several cups of this tea during the day.

To minimize the die-off effect, it is very important that the toxins are eliminated from the body as quickly as possible. Psyllium seeds are helpful in this because they swell in the gut and bind the toxins. The swelling of the seeds stimulates bowel movements, thus aiding the elimination of toxins via the faeces. You will need to take 1 to 2 tablespoons of seeds per day, sprinkled over yoghurt, muesli or salads, etc.

Another route of toxin elimination is via the kidneys. Celery seed tea acts as a gentle diuretic and helps to eliminate toxins via the kidneys. Drinking plenty of water will flush the kidneys and facilitate this process.

Don't forget that the skin is a major route of toxin elimination, and so saunas and Epsom salt baths are also very useful.

How Long Will It Take to Get Well?

The Candida regime is a difficult one, there is no doubt of that, and many people fall off the path to health because they feel that they are chained to this frugal lifestyle for ever.

First of all, you must realize that you are *not* bound by the rules of the treatment programme for ever, but you might need to be careful with your lifestyle from now on. I have found that, on average, people can feel dreadful during the first two weeks as they adapt to the treatment programme, get their shopping list in order, and go through the die-off effect. After this initial period, most people gradually start to feel better, and after three months do feel a definite improvement in their symptoms. After six months they are significantly better, and after a year most people are quite well again and very well aware of the things which make them feel good or bad.

Below is a rough guide outlining the average length of time taken for the various aspects of the treatment programme to take effect:

Healing a leaky gut	3 months
Killing the fungus	3 months or more, depending on how severe the case is
Repopulating the gut flora	6 – 8 weeks
Rebalancing your hormones	At least 4 months
Eliminating food sensitivities	At least 3 months
Rebuilding your immune system	6 –12 months, or more if you are very depleted

Remaining on the Diet

You will probably always need to keep a close eye on your diet. This is not to say that you can never enjoy chocolate or wine again, but you may find that these 'treats' make you feel so ill that you lose the urge to indulge. However, as time passes and you find yourself firmly on the path of health, you will find that you can enjoy the forbidden fruits and get away with it as long as you keep these indulgences as occasional treats. Enjoy your Christmas trifle, and have a glass of wine when you go out to dinner, but keep these treats rare.

Useful Addresses

Professional Bodies

Australia and New Zealand
Australian National Therapists Association
1 800 817577
www.anta.com.au

Allergy Association
PO Box 298
Ringwood
Victoria 3134

New Zealand Society of Naturopaths
www.naturopath.org.nz

Canada
Association of Naturopathic Physicians of British Columbia
2042786 West 16th Avenue
Vancouver
British Columbia V6K 3C4

Ontario Naturopathic Medicine Association
60 Berl Avenue
Toronto
Ontario M8Y 3C7
(416) 503 9554

United Kingdom
Aromatherapy Organisations Council
08707 7443477

British Association of Nutritional Therapists
BCM Bant
27 Old Gloucester Street
London W4 1PP
08706 061284
www.bant.org.uk

British Wheel of Yoga
25 Jermyn Street
Sleaford
Lincolnshire NG34 7RU

Colonic International Association
Drummond Ride
Tring HP23 5DE
01442 825632

International Federation of Aromatherapists
182 Chiswick High Road
London W11PP
020 8742 2605

Institute of Allergy Therapists
Ffynnonwen
Llangwyryton
Aberystwyth
Dyfed SX23 4EY
01974 241376

The National Institute of Medical Herbalists
56 Longbrook Street
Exeter
Devon EX4 6AH
01392 426022
www.nimh.org.uk
email: nimh@ukexeter.freeserve.co.uk

The Register of Qualified Aromatherapists
www.rqa-uk.org
email: admin@rqa-uk.org

Society of Homeopaths
2 Artizan Road
Northampton NN1 4HU
01604 621400

United States of America

American Association of Naturopathic Physicians
8201 Greensboro Drive, Suite 300
Mclean, VA 22102
(703) 610 9037
www.naturopathic.org

American Holistic Medical Association
4101 Lake Boone Trail, Suite 201
Raleigh, NC 27607
(703) 556 9245
www.4woman.org

Diagnostic Laboratories

UK

Biolab
Stone House
9 Weymouth Street
London W1N 3FF
020 7636 5959 only on doctor referral

Bio-Screen Ltd
Broadway House
14 Mount Pleasant Road
Tunbridge Wells
Kent TN1 1QU

Individual Wellbeing Diagnostic Laboratories
1 Cadogan Gardens
London SW3 2RJ
020 7730 7010
Fax: 020 7730 7447
www.iwdl.net
email: info@iwdl.net

York Nutritional Laboratory
Tudor House
Lysander Close
Clifton Moor
York YO3 4XB
01904 690640

US
Great Smokies Diagnostic Laboratories
63 Zillicoa Street
Ashevilla, NC 28801
1 800 5224762
www.gsoll.com

DiagnosTech
6620 South 192nd Place
Building J
Kent, WA 98032
1 800 8783787
www.diagnostechs.com

Nutritional and Herbal Suppliers
UK

Biocare
Lakeside
180 Lifford Lane
Kings Norton
Birmingham B30 3NU
0121 433 3727
Fax: 0121 433 8705

Lamberts Healthcare Ltd
1 Lamberts Road
Tunbridge Wells
Kent TN2 3EH
01892 554313
Fax: 01892 515863

Support Groups

UK

Action Against Allergy
2426 High Street
Hampton Hill
MiddlesexTW12 1TD

Action for ME and Chronic Fatigue
PO Box 1302
Wells
Somerset BA5 2WE

ME Association
PO Box 8
Stanford-le-Hope
Essex SS17 8EX

National Candida Society
PO Box 151
Orpington
Kent BR5 1UJ
www.candida-society.org.uk
email: info@candida-society.org.uk

Further Reading

Cookbooks

Beat Candida Cookbook	Erica White (Thorsons)
Cooking for Candida	Jo Hampton (Kingston House Publishing)
The Candida Diet Book	Karen Brody (Sheldon Press)

INDEX